CEREBROVASCULAR RESEARCH AND DISORDERS SERIES

HYPERTENSION, HEREDITY AND STROKE

Cerebrovascular Research and Disorders Series

Hypertension, Heredity and Stroke
Cristina Moratinos and Bruno Cárdenas
2009 ISBN: 978-1-60741-496-4

CEREBROVASCULAR RESEARCH AND DISORDERS SERIES

HYPERTENSION, HEREDITY AND STROKE

CRISTINA MORATINOS
AND
BRUNO CÁRDENAS
EDITORS

Nova Biomedical Books
New York

For permission to use material from this book please contact us:
Telephone 631-231-7269; Fax 631-231-8175
Web Site: http://www.novapublishers.com

Library of Congress Cataloging-in-Publication Data

Hypertension, heredity, and stroke / [edited by] Cristina Moratinos and Bruno Cárdenas.
p. ; cm.
Includes bibliographical references and index.
ISBN 978-1-60741-496-4 (hardcover)
1. Cerebrovascular disease in children. 2. Cerebrovascular disease. 3. Hypertension in children. 4. Hypertension. I. Moratinos, Cristina. II. Cárdenas, Bruno.
[DNLM: 1. Hypertension. 2. Adolescent. 3. Child. 4. Stroke--genetics. WG 340 H9951045 2009]
RJ496.C45H97 2009
618.92'81--dc22 2009023562

Published by Nova Science Publishers, Inc. ✝ New York

Contents

Preface **vii**

Chapter 1 Genetics of Intracerebral Hemorrhage **1**
Alessandro Pezzini, Elisabetta Del Zotto, Alessia Giossi, Irene Volonghi and Alessandro Padovani

Chapter 2 Primary Arterial Hypertension in Obese Children as a Risk Factor of the Development of Premature Atherosclerosis **25**
Maria Hanna Kniażewska and Anna Karolina Obuchowicz

Chapter 3 On the Existing Relationships between the Physical Activity, Tobacco Consumption, Body Composition and Socioeconomic Status as a Function of the Blood Pressure smong Spanish Adolescents **45**
Cordente Martínez, A. Carlos, García Soidán Pilar, Sillero Quintana, Manuel, Stirling James

Chapter 4 Ambulatory Blood Pressure Monitoring in Children with Glomerular Kidney Disease **69**
Piotr Skrzypczyk, Małgorzata Panczyk-Tomaszewska, Iwona Bieroza and Maria Roszkowska-Blaim

Chapter 5 Surgical Palliative Options for Patients with Hypoplastic Left Heart **87**
Clifford L. Cua, Christopher L. Cua and Lillian S. Lai

Chapter 6 Influence of Heart Rate on Development of Stroke among Patients at Risk for Cerebrovascular Disease **101**
Basil N. Okeahialam and Ayuba I. Zoakah

Chapter 7 Standards and Pitfalls Regarding the SHR Model in Genetic Hypertension and Stroke **113**
Hiroshi Yao and Toru Nabika

Chapter 8 Hypertensive Children Have Lower Bone Mass than Normotensive Children **125**
Afrooz Afghani

Chapter 9	Hypertension and Obesity *Alfonso D. Torres and Colette A. Gushurst*	**137**
Chapter 10	Arterial Hypertension in Children after the Surgical Repair of Aortic Coarctation *Tomasz Florianczyk, Bozena Werner, Jacek Skiendzielewski and Piotr Wieniawski*	**147**
Chapter 11	Problems of Methodology and Interpretation of Ambulatory Blood Pressure Monitoring in Children *Tomasz Florianczyk and Bozena Werner*	**157**
Chapter 12	Genetic Studies in Pediatric Stroke *Natasa Marcun Varda and Alojz Gregoric*	**163**
Index		**173**

Preface

This book gathers the latest research from around the world on hypertension and stroke. While it is widely known how raised heart rate adversely affects ischaemic heart disease and congestive heart failure, it has not been clearly shown how low heart rate increases tendency to stroke. Thus the influence of heart rate on development of stroke is examined in this book. The etiology of pediatric stroke, a potentially devastating condition, is also discussed, since it is an important condition that often remains unknown in a considerable number of patients. Furthermore, arterial hypertension and cardiovascular complications in patients with glomerular kidney disease are also explored in this book.

The progress that has been made towards identifying the genetics of risk factors in polygenic and multifactorial intracerebral hemorrhage (ICH) is presented and data regarding monogenic conditions associated with ICH is summarized. Other chapters in this book include the examination of the association between blood pressure (BP) and bone mineral content (BMC) in pediatrics; arterial hypertension as one of the main clinical symptoms of aortic coarctation in children, and a review of ambulatory blood pressure monitoring (ABPM) as a noninvasive method of blood pressure assessment, which is considered to be a very useful tool in the diagnosis of arterial hypertension in adults, teenagers and children.

Chapter 1 - The worldwide incidence of intracerebral hemorrhage (ICH) ranges from 10 to 20 cases per 100,000 population, and increases with age, although not as steeply as cerebral infarction. This figure is expected to double during the next 50 years as a result of the increasing age of the population and changes in racial demographics. There are many possible factors associated with ICH, sometimes acting alone, but most often in various combinations. Risk factors include blood vessel malformation, such as an arteriovenous malformations or aneurysms, disorders of the coagulation, or structural changes of the blood vessel wall due to hypertension or amyloid.

Many of these risk factors have a genetic background. Actually, the disease frequency varies by race and ethnicity, being more prevalent in Japanese, blacks and Hispanic individuals. Family studies also have shown an association between ICH and a positive family history of ICH, suggesting an underlying genetic etiology. The genetic risk factors for ICH are often divided into single-gene disorders, polygenic disorders (where multiple genes act together to result in certain phenotype), or multifactorial disorders (in which genetic and environmental factors may interact).

In this chapter the authors will review progress that has been made towards identifying the genetics of risk factors in polygenic and multifactorial ICH and summarize present data regarding monogenic conditions associated with ICH.

Chapter 2 - Primary arterial hypertension (HT) in children occurs significantly more often than once assumed. It is the main form of HT in children over 12 years old and is prevalent in the obese. It has been proved that birth weight influences the blood pressure development during the developmental age. According to recent data the percentage of overweight and obese children is rising drastically. It has been proved that the weight gain is accompanied by the increase in blood pressure (1 mmHg per each kilogram gained). Impaired glucose tolerance, disturbances of lipid metabolism, increase in cardiac output, sympathetic and rennin-angiotensin-aldosterone systems' activation, sodium and water retention are caused by excessive development of fatty tissue (especially visceral fat), and these factors support development of HT and early atheromatous lesions. Autopsy studies of children and young individuals in the Bogalusa Heart Study provided important information. Strict dependence between weight gain, systolic pressure, lipid disturbances, smoking and progression of atheromatous changes in the aorta and coronary arteries has been proven. These studies indicate occurrence of atherosclerosis in children and the young with risk factors predisposing to the development of atherosclerosis. Identification of CVD risk factors, constituting the metabolic syndrome (HT and obesity are integral parts of this syndrome) in children, is a subject of numerous currently performed researches. In the recent years researches have shown that adipocytes display significant endocrine and paracrine activity. Biologically active substances (influencing blood pressure regulation) secreted by these cells include among others: leptin, adiponectin, Agouti protein, visfatin, resistin, as well as TGF-β, TNF-α, PAI-1, angiotensinogen, rennin, convertase of the angiotensin, chimase, DIG catepsine, prostaglandin, IGF-1, VEGF, MIF, IL-6, sex hormones (testosterone, estradiol, estrone), glicocortycosteroids. Damage of arterial endothelium and oxidative modification of LDL molecules initiate the atheromatous process. Long-term increase in blood pressure is associated with mechanical injuries of the endothelium. The so-called shear stress, resulting from blood flow, leads to secondary activation of inflammatory process intensifying the atheromatosis. Diagnostics of HT causes in obese children with consideration of factors supporting the development of atherosclerosis (standard HT diagnostics, diagnostic of blood vessel conditions – IMT and vessel vasodilatation capability, evaluation of lipid metabolism and the level of glucose utilization and plasma antioxidant capability, evaluation of the so-called new CVD risk factors – levels of homocysteine, CRP, prothrombotic factors) is currently of great significance in primary CVD prophylaxis. Pharmacotherapy, but most importantly non-pharmacological methods of treatment aiming to modify the lifestyle (weight loss, increase in physical activity, dietary conduct, quitting smoking) are of specific significance in obese children suffering from HT.

Chapter 3 - After obtaining a written consent of the parents, subjects from ages 13 to 17 were studied in a representative sample of 474 subjects, 204 boys and 270 girls from 35 educative centres (18 privates and 17 publics) from 16 of the 21 districts of the city of Madrid.

It was found that 12.7% of the boys and 35.6% of the girls were inactive or sedentary. The socioeconomic status significantly determined the physical activity of the girls, especially in the age group 16-17. The girls had a tobacco consumption significantly superior to the boys. A significant inverse relation of the tobacco consumption with the physical activity was found for boys. 47.4% of the girls of the sample were lightly overweight to obese as opposed to the 14.7% of boys. A significant association between adiposity and physical activity in the girls was observed.

The averages for the systolic/diastolic blood pressure were 125.6/71.3 mmHg in boys and 118/69.4 mmHg in girls. A significant relation between the gender and the systolic blood pressure was found.

Solely one relation was found between the blood pressure and the others studied variables: the relation between the physical activity and the diastolic blood pressure for boys (69.9 mmHg for active or very active and 74.1 mmHg for moderately active to sedentary).

As a result of our observations the following series of proposals for the future were made:

The lack of existing relations between the blood pressure and the others variables support the hypothesis that the the effects of these variables on the cardiovascular risk factors needs a longer term to be obvious. Then, it seems to be necessary to suggest future longitudinal studies to know exactly the influence of the healthy habits on the blood pressure of children and adolescents.

Furthermore, girls and subjects from the lower socioeconomico status should receive high-priority attention concerning the health-related habits as physical activity, tobacco consumption or dietary habits which could have a great influence in the future on the blood pressure and other cardiovascular risk factors.

Chapter 4 - INTRODUCTION: Arterial hypertension and cardiovascular complications are common problems in patients with glomerulonephritis. Ambulatory blood pressure monitoring (ABPM) is a useful method for early evaluation of hypertension.

PURPOSE OF THE STUDY: The purpose of the study was to analyze ABPM parameters and to evaluate its usefulness in the evaluation of arterial hypertension in children with glomerular kidney disease.

MATERIAL AND METHODS: The study involved 47 children aged 4.5 to 18 (mean 14.2+3.3) years, including 17 patients with IgA nephropathy or Schoenlein-Henoch syndrome, 9 with idiopathic nephrotic syndrome, and 22 with other forms of glomerulonephritis. ABPM was performed in all children. The following ABPM parameters were analyzed: systolic, diastolic and mean blood pressure during 24 hrs (sBP/24h, dBP/24h, MAP/24h), activity (sBP/a, dBP/a, MAP/a) and resting period (sBP/r, dBP/r, MAP/r); systolic and diastolic blood pressure load during 24 hrs (sBPL/24h, dBPL/24h), activity (sBPL/a, dBPL/a) and resting period (sBPL/r, dBPL/r); pulse pressure (PP) during 24 hrs (PP/24h), activity (PP/a) and resting period (PP/r); and circadian blood pressure profile and systolic and diastolic blood pressure index during 24 hrs (sBPI/24, dBPI/24), activity (sBPI/a, dBPI/a) and resting period (sBPI/r, dBPI/r). Renal function (serum creatinine level, estimated GFR according to the Schwartz formula), proteinuria, and the use of antihypertensive, renoprotective, and immunosuppressive treatment were analyzed in all children.

RESULTS: Based on ABPM, hypertension could be diagnosed in 17 patients (36%). Among 30 patients without hypertension in ABPM, six (20%) had elevated (>25%) blood pressure load during 24 hrs, and in another six (20%) elevated blood pressure load was only found during the resting period. Elevated PP was found in 24 (51%) patients. Disturbed circadian blood pressure rhythm was observed in 13 (28%) patients. Proteinuria [mg/kg/24h] correlated positively with sBPI/24h, dBPI/24h, sBPI/a, sBPI/r, dBPI/a, dBPI/r, sBPL/24h, dBPL/24h, sBPL/a, sBPL/r, dBPL/a and dBPL/r. Prednisone doses [mg/kg/24h] correlated positively with sBPI/24h, dBPI/24h, sBPI/a, sBPI/r, dBPI/a, dBPI/r, sBPL/24h, dBPL/24h, sBPL/a, dBPL/a, sBPL/r, and dBPL/r.

CONCLUSIONS: ABPM is a useful method in the evaluation of arterial hypertension in children with various forms of glomerulonephritis. Arterial hypertension, disturbed circadian rhythm of blood pressure and elevated pulse pressure are common findings in children with glomerulonephritis. Higher blood pressure parameters were seen in ABPM in children with more severe proteinuria and in children taking higher prednisone doses.

Chapter 5- Hypoplastic left heart syndrome (HLHS) was once considered a lethal condition with the two treatment options consisting of hospice care or transplantation; however, with the advent of surgical palliation, first described by Norwood, morbidity and mortality has steadily improved for this patient population. In the current era, three surgical palliations are possible for the initial procedure. These options include: 1) Norwood procedure with pulmonary blood flow supplied via a modified Blalock-Taussig shunt, 2) modification of the Norwood procedure with pulmonary blood flow supplied with a right ventricle to pulmonary artery conduit, or 3) hybrid procedure consisting of bilateral pulmonary artery banding, ductus arteriosus stenting, and balloon atrial septostomy. Each method has certain advantages and disadvantages that make them unique. No method at this time has proven consistently superior and it may be that each procedure has certain advantages over the other depending on the clinical situation and HLHS anatomy. The authors review the current literature for the three surgical variations with the goal of obtaining a better understanding of the possible surgical options for this complex disease.

Chapter 6 - Background: The importance of heart rate as a prognostic factor and potential therapeutic target, despite suggestive evidence has not yet been generally accepted. Whereas drugs that reduce heart rate improve outcome in ischaemic heart disease and congestive cardiac failure, such is said not to be the experience with stroke. It has been reported that uncomplicated hypertension treated with beta blockers is associated with an increase in stroke especially in the elderly. While it is known how raised heart rate adversely affects ischaemic heart disease and congestive cardiac failure, it has not been clearly shown how low heart rate increases tendency to stroke. This report is on studies which suggest that lower heart rate is related to the occurrence of stroke.

Methods: Two cohorts of stroke patients had their heart rates determined clinically. Drugs and diseases likely to affect heart rate served as exclusion criteria. Finally only those in sinus rhythm were enrolled. They were compared with sex and age (+ 5 years) matched controls on who the same criteria applied along three lines: mean values, proportions along above and below average heart rate lines; as well as in six different heart rate groups. Pair-matched analysis of data was also done.

Results: In the first cohort, the mean heart rate of 77.5 + 13.3 per minute was significantly lower than the mean of 90.3 + 13.6 per minute among the controls ($t = 3.17$. $p< 0.01$). Along the lines of above and below average, the proportion of stroke patients whose heart rates was below average was significantly higher than the controls (chi square with

Yates correction = 4.17. $p < 0.05$). When grouped into six, the proportions of the cases was significantly higher than the controls in classes < 60/minute ($t = 2.06$. $p < 0.05$) and 61 – 70/minute ($t = 2.14$. $p < 0.05$). For the class >100/minute, the cases were significantly fewer than the controls ($t = 2.26$. $p < 0.05$).

In the second cohort, the mean heart rate of 78.4 + 10.4 per minute among cases was lower than, but not significantly from 82.3 + 8.4 per minute recorded for the controls. However when grouped above or below average, the proportion of stroke patients below average was significantly higher than controls (chi square with Yates correction = 9.08. $p < 0.01$). Along the six group lines, significant difference emerged only in the 61 – 70/minute range, with cases more than controls ($t = 4.38$. $p < 0.0001$).

When pair-matched analysis was done using McNemars's test, the association between stroke cases and low heart rate was highly significant ($p < 0.001$)

Discussion: The lower the heart rate, the more sluggish the circulation. This makes for thrombus formation especially as the arterial tree may have been narrowed from atherosclerotic plaques caused by predisposing diseases. Consequently the chances of ischaemic stroke from thrombo-embolism would be raised especially during periods of inactivity.

Chapter 7 - Spontaneously hypertensive rats (SHR) was developed by Okamoto and Aoki (1963) by selective inbreedings from the Wistar-Kyoto rats (WKY). SHR are relevant to stroke research and are used widely for studies of hypertension-related cerebraovascular complications. However, one of the most annoying problems with using SHR in stroke research is that SHR or its normotensive control WKY from different sources are genetically heterogeneous. SHR/Izm have emerged as a prototype of SHR, which are derived from original SHR. The SHRSP was originally established from the A substrain of the SHR, and two other substrains of SHR, the B and C substrains, are stroke resistant. B substrain corresponds to SHR/Izm.

The authors have established a focal ischemia model utilizing the laser system (photothrombotic distal middle cerebral artery [MCA] occlusion and YAG laser induced reperfusion). Photothrombotic occlusion of distal MCA in SHR provides a simple and reproducible model of stroke or focal ischemia. A congenic strategy using inbred rat strains that display genetic hypertension (i.e., SHR) is a powerful method by which to examine the effects of polygenic traits on the stroke phenotype. Recently, they examined the effects of the congenic removal of a blood pressure quantitative trait locus (QTL) on stroke phenotype (i.e., infarct volume after MCA occlusion [MCAO]). Based on this experience, the authors would like to comment on the standards and pitfalls of stroke models in the research on genetic hypertension and stroke.

Chapter 8 - *Background:* The association between blood pressure (BP) and bone mineral content (BMC) has not been extensively studied in pediatrics. *Design:* Cross-sectional study. *Participants:* 187 (105 boys, 82 girls) overweight (BMI=28.7 kg/m^2) Latino children and adolescents (age=11.2 years). *Assessment of Risk Factors:* Seated systolic (SBP) and diastolic (DBP) blood pressure measured using a standard mercury sphygmomanometer. Hypertension defined by SBP or DBP above the 90th percentile for height, age, and gender. *Main Outcome Measurements:* Total body BMC measured by dual-energy x-ray absorptiometry. *Results:* There was an inverse association between SBP and BMC (r=-0.24, p=0.02) in boys; results were non-significant (p=0.27) in girls. There were no significant correlations between DBP and BMC in either boys or girls. Hypertensive boys (n=21) had lower BMC (1437 versus 1639 g; p=0.02) than normotensive boys (n=84); similarly, hypertensive girls (n=25) had lower BMC (1435 versus 1620 g; p=0.01) than normotensive girls (n=57). In post-pubertal boys (Tanner stage 4-5; n=11), inverse correlations between SBP and BMC were markedly stronger (r=-0.80, p=0.02). *Conclusion:* SBP is inversely correlated with BMC in overweight adolescents, with the strongest association observed in adolescent boys. Additionally, hypertensives have lower adjusted means of BMC than normotensives. Hypertension may be a risk factor for osteopenia in overweight children and adolescents.

Chapter 9 - The link between obesity and hypertension is examined in this chapter. Underlying mechanisms include increase in sympathetic activity, sodium balance, renal tubular sodium reabsorption, glomerular filtration rate (GFR) and development of insulin resistance. The role of leptin is examined in the development of hypertension in obese adolescents. Also considered in this review are the definitions of hypertension and principles of management for obese youth with hypertension. Pharmacologic agents used for management of hypertension include diuretics, alpha blockers, beta blockers, angiotensin converting enzyme inhibitors (ACE inhibitors), angiotensin-2 receptor blockers (ARBs), and long acting calcium channel blockers. The importance of weight control, caloric restriction, and exercise in the management of obesity in youth is also stressed.

Chapter 10 - Arterial hypertension is one of main clinical symptoms of aortic coarctation in children and could be also observed after the surgical treatment despite of good result of the surgery.

The prevalence of arterial hypertension in children successfully treated due to coarctation of the aorta ranges from 7% to 75% according to various authors. The risk of arterial hypertension rises with the patient's age and follow-up period after surgery. Moreover the incidence of postcoarctectomy hypertension is quite low in children operated in infancy in comparison to these who undergo surgical treatment in older age.

Arterial hypertension could be observed immediately after the surgical treatment as a result of sympathetic nervous system hyperstymulation due to baroreceptor reflex or increased activity of the complex of rennin-angiotensin–aldosteron. The authors observed a hypertension crisis in infant just after the balloon angioplasty of aortic recoarctation who underwent the procedure 4 months after the primary surgical treatment.

In etiology of late postcoarctectomy hypertension the following factors are considered: residual aortic coarctation, decreased sensitivity of baroreceptor reflex, increased activity of the rennin-angiotensin-aldosteron complex and rise of vasopressin secretion.

In evaluated group of 93 patients after the successful surgical repair of aortic coarctation hypertension was found in 24,7% of cases based on sphygmomanometer measurement and in 19,3% of cases using ABPM. In children operated in infancy the prevalence was 11,4 %, while in those operated in older age 34,4%.

Chapter 11 - Ambulatory blood pressure monitoring (ABPM) is a noninvasive method of blood pressure assessment commonly found as a useful tool in diagnosis of arterial hypertension in adults, teenagers and children.

For the last 11 years the authors have collected about 2000 ABPM recordings performed in children and adolescents. Although the authors have found ABPM as a very valuable method, the authors need to point out some important drawbacks such as: lack of standardization of recording protocol and specification of commonly acceptable normal ranges and rules of interpretation.

The authors perform ABPM recordings in children older than six years of age. In our opinion in these patients measurements are well tolerated, moreover the number of artifacts is small enough to qualify majority of the recordings for further analysis. Our own protocol of ABPM includes repetition of measurements every 30 minutes in daytime and 60 minutes in nighttime in the youngest patients (6 and 7 years old) and adequately every 15 and 30 minutes in older children. The authors believe that values of mean systolic and mean diastolic blood pressure calculated for all of 24 hours period are crucial parameters to confirm or exclude the suspicion of arterial hypertension. Nevertheless there are still some doubts how to interpret blood pressure load and nocturnal deep. The authors diagnose the arterial hypertension in all of those patients whose blood pressure load exceeds 25%. Children with nocturnal fall lower than 10% are qualified as a non-dippers for further observation. In contrast to a standard blood pressure measurement there are still no commonly used normal ranges. This makes a main limitation of ABPM.

Thus the authors postulate to prepare commonly acceptable rules of protocol standardization as well as an interpretation of recordings with a special attention to blood pressure load. The tables of ABPM normal ranges for various ethnic groups and countries should be worked out.

Chapter 12 - Cerebrovascular diseases in children are a heterogeneous group of disorders with both genetic and environmental etiological factors. Despite extensive investigation, the etiology of pediatric stroke, a potentially devastating condition, remains unknown in a considerable number of patients. In recent years, progress in the field of molecular genetics has enabled research into genetic factors. In addition, the importance of classifying stroke subtypes in children has been ascertained.

In our opinion, besides children suffering from strokes, the children of parents with premature stroke represent an important group for research into genetic factors, since early manifestations of a severe cerebrovascular event generally indicate a strong genetic basis for the disorder. Additionally, in young patients, the role of environmental factors (e.g. diet, smoking) is relatively less important. On the other hand, because of the complex nature of the disease, environmental factors have to be studied simultaneously, possibly with some of the methods enabling detection of early and subclinical manifestations of the disease process.

Furthermore, environmental exposure (e.g. infection, hypoxemia) may play a crucial role in modifying genetic expression and hence it must be carefully defined.

In light of the above, the authors performed a pilot study of some genetic and environmental factors in children of patients with a documented cerebrovascular accident before the age of 45 years and looked for carotid artery intima-media thickness, which represents a marker of early vascular disease.

In the future, a larger sample of these children should be studied, with careful classification of stroke and control of environmental factors. Genetic factors related to atherosclerosis and thrombosis, as well as the interaction between these factors and the role of possible environmental modifiers, should be investigated. The authors plan to undertake such a study in the near future. The same research principle should be used in children who have suffered a stroke.

In: Hypertension, Heredity and Stroke
Editor: Cristina Moratinos and Bruno Cardenas
ISBN 978-1-60741-496-4

Chapter 1

Genetics of Intracerebral Hemorrhage

***Alessandro Pezzini*[*1], *Elisabetta Del Zotto*[2], *Alessia Giossi*[1], *Irene Volonghi*[1] *and Alessandro Padovani*[1]**

[1]Dipartimento di Scienze Mediche e Chirurgiche, Clinica Neurologica, Università degli Studi di Brescia, Brescia, Italia

[2]Dipartimento di Scienze Biomediche e Biotecnologie, Università degli Studi di Brescia, Brescia, Italia

Abstract

The worldwide incidence of intracerebral hemorrhage (ICH) ranges from 10 to 20 cases per 100,000 population, and increases with age, although not as steeply as cerebral infarction. This figure is expected to double during the next 50 years as a result of the increasing age of the population and changes in racial demographics. There are many possible factors associated with ICH, sometimes acting alone, but most often in various combinations. Risk factors include blood vessel malformation, such as an arteriovenous malformations or aneurysms, disorders of the coagulation, or structural changes of the blood vessel wall due to hypertension or amyloid.

Many of these risk factors have a genetic background. Actually, the disease frequency varies by race and ethnicity, being more prevalent in Japanese, blacks and Hispanic individuals. Family studies also have shown an association between ICH and a positive family history of ICH, suggesting an underlying genetic etiology. The genetic risk factors for ICH are often divided into single-gene disorders, polygenic disorders (where multiple genes act together to result in certain phenotype), or multifactorial disorders (in which genetic and environmental factors may interact).

In this chapter we will review progress that has been made towards identifying the genetics of risk factors in polygenic and multifactorial ICH and summarize present data regarding monogenic conditions associated with ICH.

[*] Tel: +39.030.399 5631 – 5632; Fax: +39.030.399 5027, e-mail: ale_pezzini@hotmail.com

Abbreviations

ICH	intracerebral hemorrhage
PICH	primary intracerebral hemorrhage
CAA	cerebral amyloid angiopathy
CMMs	cerebral cavernous malformations (cerebral cavernous hemangiomas)
AVMs	arteriovenous malformations
TIAs	transient ischemic attacks
MRI	magnetic resonance imaging
APP	amyloid precursor protein
AD	Alzheimer's disease
HCHWA-D	hereditary cerebral hemorrhage with amyloidosis Dutch type
HCHWA-I	hereditary cerebral amyloid with amyloidosis Icelandic type
APOE	apolipoprotein E
CAAH	cerebral amyloid angiopathy-related hemorrhage
FXIII	factor XIII
FV	factor V
FII,	factor II
FVII	factor VII
PAF	platelet-activating factor
TUBB1	β1-tubulin
ACT	anti-chymotrypsin
TGFβ	transforming growth factor-beta
ENG	endoglin
HHT	hereditary hemorragic teleangiectasia
ACE	angiotensin converting enzyme
ALK1	activin receptor-like kinase 1
KRIT1	Krev interaction trapped 1

Introduction

Intracerebral hemorrhage (ICH) is defined as a bleeding into the parenchima of the brain that may extend into the ventricles and, in rare cases, into the subarachnoid space.

ICH accounts for 10 to 15 % of all cases of stroke and is associated with the highest mortality rate, with only 38 % of affected patients surviving the first year [1]. The worldwide incidence of ICH has been estimated to range from 10 to 20 cases per 100,000 population and to increase with age [2]. As a consequence of the increasing age of the population and changes in racial demographics this figure is expected to double during the next 50 years. Intraparenchymal bleeding results from the rupture of an abnormally formed vessel, as in the case of a vascular malformations, or from a vessel damaged by a chronic or acute pathologic process.

Notwithstanding, only 20% of ICHs have a clear cause of arterial rupture identified on brain imaging or cerebral angiography [3,4]. Therefore, the cause of ICH is not immediately clear in most cases. Sometimes a specific cause can be suggested by the age of the patient, the use of medication and previous medical history in combination with neuroimaging features, such as localization, size and form of the hemorrhage, and its association with other structural abnormalities.

Based on the underlying cause of the vessel rupture, ICH is traditionally classified as *primary* or *secondary*. Primary intracerebral hemorrhage (PICH), defined as a hemorrhage within the parenchyma in the absence of readily identifiable causes, is the prevalent type, accounting for 78 to 88 % of cases. In spite of this definition PICH can not be considered a random event, but rather the result of a specific underlying vascular process such as hypertensive vasculopathy or the increasingly recognized entity of cerebral amyloid angiopathy (CAA). Secondary ICH is defined as a hemorrhage resulting from trauma, rupture of vascular abnormalities, coagulopathy or other causes [2].

Table 1. Main causes of intracerebral haemorrhage

Main causes
Hypertension
Amyloid angiopathy
Arterio-venous malformations
Cavernous hemangiomas
Intracranial aneurysms
Intracranial neoplasms
Primary or metastatic tumors
Coagulopathies
Hereditary coagulopathies
Leukemia, DIC
Thrombocytopenia and other platelet disorders
Hepatic and renal failure
Antithrombotic medications use
Dural venous sinus thrombosis
Vasculitis
Illicit drugs
Cocaine, heroin, ecstasy
Alcohol use
Hemorrhagic ischemic stroke
Head traumas

Cerebral arteriovenous malformations (AVMs), cavernous hemangiomas (CMMs) or aneurysms represent the most common vascular abnormalities associated with the occurrence of ICH. Coagulopathies can be the consequence of medication use as well as of hereditary disorders of hemostasis.

ICH commonly occurs in the cerebral lobes, basal ganglia, thalamus, brain stem (predominantly the pons), and cerebellum. On the basis of the location of bleeding, ICH is classified as *lobar* (when occurring in lobar brain regions) and *non-lobar* (when involving deep hemispheric structures). Different pathogenic mechanisms are presumed to underline these two entities. Similarly, the rate of recurrence has suggested to be different in these ICH subtypes, the risk being higher for lobar than for non-lobar ICH [5].

Most of the risk factors for ICH have a genetic background. Furthermore, data on the biologic mechanisms underlying the pathologic conditions related to ICH, in particular CAA, have given important clues in defining potential genetic risk factors for ICH.

In this chapter we will review progress that has been made in the identification of the genetics of ICH and summarize data on specific monogenic conditions associated with ICH.

Risk Factors for ICH

There are many possible risk factors associated with ICH, some of them acting alone, but most often in various combination [2]. The most important contributors to ICH are the presence of arterial hypertension and CAA. However, many additional factors also play a role in influencing the occurrence of ICH. Epidemiological evidence indicate that advancing age, heavy alcohol intake and anticoagulant treatment are consistently associated with ICH [4,6-9]. Although data are still conflicting, cholesterolemia, a traditional risk factor for ischemic disease, has been related to ICH with a reverse effect, the lower risk being associated with higher cholesterol levels [10].

Genetic Risk Factors

Family History as a Risk Factor for ICH

Several studies have pointed out an association between ICH and positive family history of ICH, thus providing data for a genetic basis of this condition [6,11,12]. In the population-based Cincinnati/Northern Kentucky study, Woo and colleagues found that having a first-degree relative with ICH is a strong risk factor both for lobar (OR 12; 95% CI 1.3-122) and for non-lobar ICH (OR 6.3; 95% CI 1.1-35) [6]. As opposed to ischemic stroke, data from twin studies are not available for ICH. In the Danish Twin Registry an increased risk of stroke death and stroke hospitalization in monozygotic compared with dizygotic co-twins was observed. However, the distinction between ICH and cerebral infarction was not reliable, since diagnoses recorded in that registry were found to have inadequate predictive values. Nevetheless, the Authors hypothesized that the genetic component might be stronger for hemorrhagic stroke than for ischemic stroke since the relative risk for fatal stroke, which is likely to be hemorrhagic, was greater than that for fatal and non-fatal strokes combined [13].

Specific Genetic Pathways

Over the last years, ICH, like other diseases of the central nervous system, has become increasingly accessible to genetic investigation, as a result of technologic advances in both clinical diagnosis and molecular genetics [14,15]. As a consequence of above, a better understanding of the pathophysiology of ICH has been gained, pointing toward specific genes and alleles playing a role in the pathogenesis of the disease.

Genes Associated with CAA

CAA is one of the most important contributors to spontaneous ICH, especially for lobar hemorrhage [16]. Amyloid is a term used to describe protein deposits with circumscript physical characteristics: β-pleated sheet configuration, apple green birefringence under polarized light after Congo red staining, fibrillary structure and high insolubility [17]. There are many different proteins that can accumulate as amyloid, and there are many different disease processes that can lead to amyloid formation. Several types of CAA have been identified in association with various amyloid proteins including amyloid β protein (Aβ), cystatin C, prion protein, thransthyretin, gelsolin and ABri/ADan [18,19]. In cerebral amyloid angiopathy, amyloid deposition occurs in the wall of medium- and small-sized leptomeningeal and cortical arteries, arterioles and, less frequently, capillaries and veins [20]. Amyloid deposition can weaken the vessel wall, causing rupture and lobar ICH. This process is also responsible for the obliteration of the vessel lumen leading to ischemia (cerebral infarction, "incomplete" infarction, and leucoencephalopathy). Though CAA can frequently be asymptomatic, it can also present with a spectrum of clinical presentations [18,21]. These include lobar hemorrhage, leucoencephalopathy, transient neurological events such as TIAs, seizures and migrainous phenomena due to perivascular inflammation, cognitive impairment and dementia [22,23]. Lobar hemorrhage may be multiple and recurrent in patients who survive the initial bleed.

The accepted criteria (the so called "Boston criteria") for CAA-related hemorrhage (CAAH) define 3 levels of diagnostic evidence: *definite* CAAH, *probable* CAAH (with and without supporting pathological data), and *possible* CAAH [24].

Neuropathological post-mortem confirmation is required for a definite diagnosis. The other categories require neuroimaging, ideally by use of gradient-echo magnetic resonance imaging (MRI) which is useful in accurately detecting microbleeds in the form of hemosiderin deposits in cortical and deep grey matter.

CAA occurs within a heterogeneous group of hereditary and sporadic diseases. Hereditary forms account for the minority of the CAA cases but have more pleomorphic phenotypes. Sporadic CAA increases dramatically with age, rarely being present before the age of 50, and increasing in prevalence to more than 50% in people over age 90 [23,25].

Table 2. Diagnostic criteria for Cerebral Amyloid Angiopathy (Boston Criteria) [24]

Definite CAA

Full postmortem examination demonstrating the following features:
Lobar, cortical o subcortical hemorrhage
Severe CAA†
Absence of other diagnostic lesion

Probable CAA with support of pathological data

Clinical data and pathologic tissue (obtained by evacuated hematoma or cortical biopsy) demonstrating the following features:
Lobar, cortical o subcortical hemorrhage
Some degree of CAA in hystological sample
Absence of other diagnostic lesion

Probable CAA

Clinical data and MRI demonstrating the following features:
Multiple hemorrhages restricted to lobar, cortical or subcortical regions *
Age ≥ 55 years
Absence of other causes of bleeding‡

Possible CAA

Clinical data and MRI demonstrating the following features:
Single lobar, cortical or subcortical hemorrhage without another cause, or multiple hemorrhages with a possible but not a definite cause or with some hemorrhages in an atypical location (e.g thalamus)
Age ≥ 55 years
Absence of other causes of bleeding‡

† Defined as a complete replacement of the media with focal vessel wall fragmentation and at least one microscopic focus of paravascular blood leakage [25].

* Cerebellar hemorrhage also included.

‡ Included: excessive warfarin (INR >3.0); antecedent head trauma or ischemic stroke; CNS tumor, vascular malformation or vasculitis; blood dyscrasia or coagulopathy. (INR>3.0 or other nonspecific laboratory abnormalities permitted for diagnosis of possible CAA).

The genetics of CAA have been studied for both familial and sporadic forms.

Hereditary forms of CAA are rare and account for a minority of the CAA cases [19]. Described in a single family or a small number of families, a mutated variant protein or precursor protein is abnormally metabolized by proteolitic pathways and accumulates as amyloid [17]. Hereditary CAA is characterized by a considerable heterogeneous phenotype with a large variation in age at onset, presenting symptoms, and course of the disease, which sometimes makes the diagnosis difficult.

Table 3. Hereditary cerebral amyloid angiopathy

Hereditary CAA	Amyloid protein	Gene/chromosome location	Characteristics
Hereditary cerebral hemorrhage with amyloidosis			
Dutch type (HCHWA-D)	Amyloid β protein	Mutation at codon 693 in APP gene on chromosome 21	Lobar brain hemorrhages; dementia in survivors; epilepsy in survivors; leukoencephalopathy; mean age at onset 50 years
Italian type	Amyloid β protein	Mutation at codon 693 in APP gene on chromosome 21*	Lobar brain hemorrhages and dementia
Iowa-type	Amyloid β protein	Mutation at codon 694 in APP gene on chromosome 21	Dementia; lobar brain hemorrhages (in Spanish kindred)
Flemish-type	Amyloid β protein	Mutation at codon 692 in APP gene on chromosome 20	Dementia; lobar brain hemorrhages
Icelandic-type (HCHWA-I)	Variant cystatin C	Mutation at codon 68 in cystein C gene on chromosome 20	Lobar brain hemorrhages; cognitive impairment or dementia in survivors; mean age at onset 20 years
Cerebral amyloid angiopathy in transthyretin amyloidosis	Transthyretin	Various mutation in transthyretin gene on chromosome14	Polyneuropathy; in a small number of patients ataxia, spasticity and dementia; subaracnoid hemorrhage reported
Cerebral amyloid angiopathy in prion disease	Prion protein	Mutation in PRNP gene on chromosome 13	Dementia, ataxia, extrapyramidal signs and spastic paraparesis; age of onset 40 years
Cerebral amyloid angiopathy in gelsolin amyloidosis	Gelsolin	Mutations at codon 654 in gelsolin gene on chromosome 9	Dementia; ataxia; neuropsychiatric features; corneal lattice dystrophy; cranial and peripheral neuropathy
Cerebral amyloid angiopathy in Presenilin 1 (PS-1) and Presenilin 2 (PS-2) mutations	Amyloid β protein	Mutations at codon in PS-1 gene on chromosome 14 or at codon in PS-2 gene on chromosome 1	Progressive autosomal dominant Alzheimer dementia; lobar brain hemorrhage
Familial British dementia	ABri protein	Stop codon mutation in BRI gene on chromosome 13	Dementia; spasticity; ataxia and rarely lobar intracerebral hemorrhage
Familial Danish dementia	ADan fragment protein	Decamer duplication at codon 265-266 in BRI gene on chromosome 13	Dementia; cataracts; deafness; spasticity; ataxia; rarely stroke

This phenotypic heterogeneity is probably partly caused by additional vascular risk factors, many of which are also genetically determined [26]. Most of the CAA-related mutations, with ICH as part of the clinical phenotype, involve the amyloid precursor gene, the cystatin C gene, the BRI gene and the presenilin 1 and 2 genes.

Amyloid Precursor Gene

β-amyloid peptide (Aβ) is a 39- to 43-amino acid fragment derived from the β-amyloid precursor protein (APP), encoded by a gene on chromosome 21. Aβ is proteolytically processed from APP by β- and γ-secretases. Several mutations within the Aβ sequence of APP, defined by names assigned according to the residence of the index family, are associated with autosomal dominant forms of familial CAA and include the Dutch E22Q15 mutation [27], the Italian E22K17 mutation [28], the Flemish A21G mutation [29], and the Iowa D23N mutation [30].

Each point mutation is associated with prominent CAA and hemorrhagic lesions, though Iowa [30] and Flemish [29,31] kindred show substantial Alzheimer's disease (AD) pathology as well. Among these genetic conditions, hereditary cerebral hemorrhage with amyloidosis Dutch type (HCHWA-D) is mainly characterized by ICH. HCHWA-D is a rare autosomal dominant disorder caused by a mutation at codon 693 of the APP gene, resulting in the substitution of a glutamine for a glutamic acid at position 22 of the Aβ sequence on chromosome 21 [32,33]. Almost all affected patients develop recurrent ICH and infarcts, often leading to early death [34]. Dementia can develop after the first stroke, but sometimes it is the first or the only symptom of HCHWA-D.

All CAA-related mutations fall within the Aβ region of APP, specifically at the adjacent Aβ residues 21, 22 and 23, and seem to effect Aβ fibrillogenesis, leading to excessive CAA. Mutations at Aβ positions 22 and 23 appear to generate an Aβ peptide with heightened fibrillogenic properties and increased toxicity toward components of the vessel wall [28,35-39]. The precise biochemical mechanism for the increased toxicity remains to be determined. Notwithstanding some evidence points towards a pathogenic role for the loss of the negatively charged residues [36]. By contrast, AD-associated mutations that flank the Aβ sequence, predominantly increase the relative or total amount of Aβ42 and seem to be primarily related to excessive senile plaque formation thus appearing to affect APP processing rather Aβ toxicity [40]. The Flemish mutation at Aβ position 21 also may act primarily through altered APP processing rather than increased peptide toxicity [38,39,41].

Cystatin C Gene

Familial CAA is also associated with mutation in the gene encoding cystatin C, a protease inhibitor unrelated to APP. The point mutation in exon 2 of this gene with an A→T substitution resulting in amino acid change from leucine to glutamine is responsible for the hereditary cerebral amyloid with amyloidosis Icelandic type (HCHWA-I) [42]. This is an autosomal dominant disorder causing early onset ICH and characterized by very early deposition of mutant cysteine protease inhibitor cystatin C fragment in the vessel wall. The amyloid angiopathy is more widely distribuited in this type of amyloid angiopathy than in other type and involves arteries in the cerebrum cerebellum and brainstem.

BRI Gene

Familial British dementia is another form of CAA without Aβ deposition. This condition is caused by a point mutation in the BRI gene, located on chromosome 13 [43] and clinically characterized by dementia, ataxia and rare lobar hemorrhage [44]. A single nucleotide substitution in the BRI stop codon results in the generation of an abnormal carboxyl-terminus peptide, the ABri peptide, which is deposited as amyloid fibrils in the vessel wall.

Presenilin 1 and 2 Genes

Mutations also have been identified in presenilin 1 and 2, two related genes associated with familial AD and altered processing of APP. A pedigree with mutant presenilin 2 has been reported in which patients show advanced CAA and at least one family member with hemorrhagic stroke [45]. Recently hemorrhagic strokes have also been described in a Spanish family with a novel mutation in exon 8 of the presenilin 1 gene (L286P) associated with early-onset autosomal dominant AD and lobar hematomas [46].

Sporadic CAA

Sparse reports suggest that genes associated with hereditary CAA do not play a major role as risk factors for sporadic disease. The cystatin C Icelandic mutation has been reported in only one case in sporadic CAA patients described in the literature [47-49]. Similarly, searches for APP mutations at positions 22 or 23 have yielded no instances in 111 reported sporadic CAA patients [47].

Apolipoprotein E

Among the polymorphisms associated with an increased risk for sporadic CAA-related hemorrhage (CAAH), the apolipoprotein E (APOE) genotypes have received particular attention and have been intensively studied, though with contradicting results.

The protein product apoE is a glycoprotein with three common isoforms, E2, E3, and E4, encoded by the alleles ε2, ε3, and ε4, giving rise to six genotypes, with the genotype ε3/ ε3 occurring in about one half to two thirds of people in most populations. Previously identified as a risk factor for dyslipidemia and AD, the apolipoprotein E genotypes are likely to have a role in the pathogenesis of sporadic CAA, which is thought to account for a substantial proportion of lobar ICHs in the elderly. Possible explanations for the link between APOE and

CAAH come from the evidence of a strong association between CAA with dementia and AD. In one of the largest series with pathological verification of CAAH one third of the patients had a previous history of dementia [50]. Patients with CAAH not only have the expected excess of APO ε4 allele [51-53], correlating with AD and CAA [54], but also have an over-representation of the APOE ε2 allele [52,55], which is known to be protective against AD. In particular, McCarron and Nicoll found a significant association between the APO ε2 allele and CAAH among both subjects with and without AD, whereas the APO ε4-CAAH relation correlated with concomitant AD [56]. These data provide evidence for a role of APO ε2 as a specific risk factor for CAAH, while APO ε4 seems to be non-specifically related to CAA. Furthermore, the two APOE alleles appear not only to increase the risk for CAA but also to lower the age of first hemorrhage [51] and to increase the risk of early recurrence [52]. More recently, controversial findings have been reported about the role of APOE ε4 and some studies were unable to confirm the association between the APOE ε4 allele and lobar ICH [55,57]. A recent meta-analysis of the studies which analyzed the relationship between APOE and ICH showed a significant association for the ε2-carriers (OR 1,32; 95% CI 1,01 to 1,74), with a stronger effect for lobar hemorrhages (OR 2,37; 95% CI 1,45 to 3,87). By contrast, a non-significant trend toward an association for the ε4-carriers was observed, and still a non-significant and more relevant relationship with lobar hemorrhage than with deep hemorrhage [58]. How the two APOE alleles may influence the risk of CAA-related hemorrhage is not clear and different hypotheses have been made. The ε4 allele seems to enhance amyloid deposition in blood vessels [53,54]. Conversely, the ε2 allele appears to promote degenerative changes, such as cracking and fibrinoid necrosis, leading to rupture of amyloid laden vessels [59,23]. The observation that the rare APOE ε4/ε2 genotype is associated with a particularly severe disease course [52,23] further supports the assumption that APO ε4 and ε2 have complementary roles in CAA progression.

Genes Associated with Hemostasis

Disturbances of coagulation, both iatrogenic or less frequently due to hereditary conditions, are an important cause of ICH, representing up to 8% of all cases [60,61]. Of these, the use of anticoagulant medications is the most frequent cause [8,62-64]. Moreover there is emerging evidence that anticoagulant [50,65] and possibly antiplatelet therapy [50] may be associated with a greater risk of ICH in patients with CAA than in patients without. The magnitude of such a risk seems to be higher among APOE ε2-carriers [50,65]. Hereditary disorders of hemostasis are less frequent causes of ICH [60,66]. Various genetic clotting factor deficiencies can result in intracerebral bleeding. ICH is the leading cause of death in patients with fibrinogen deficiencies, and the cause of death in many patients with hemophilia A (factor VIII deficiency), and hemophilia B (factor IX deficiency). Patients with factor VII, X, V, XI and XIII deficiencies can also suffer from ICH. Cases have been also described in patients with platelet disorders such as congenital magakaryocyte hypoplasia and the Wiskott-Aldrich syndrome [66]. In sickle cell disease ICH can occur in patients with prior infarction, due to Moya-Moya disease or aneurysmal dilatation in the region of intimal hyperplasia [67]. Information regarding history of previous hemorrhagic events, either spontaneous or associated with dental procedures, and detailed family history are important clues in suspected hematological causes of ICH. Searching for the presence of petechiae, ecchymoses and hepatosplenomegaly on physical examination is also of outstanding relevance.

Association Studies

The relation between ICH and coagulation disturbances supports the possibility that genetic variability in the hemostatic system may influence the likelihood of sporadic ICH. Relatively few studies have investigated the relationship between ICH and polymorphisms in coagulation factors, and, to date, no robust relationship has been established.

Factor XIII

Among coagulation factors, the genetic influence of the factor XIII (FXIII) on ICH has been intensively investigated. FXIII is a transglutaminase with a key role in the cross–linking of fibrin and other plasma proteins and, thus, in clot formation. Inherited deficiency of coagulation FXIII is a very rare autosomal-recessive bleeding disorder characterized by a high rate of ICH. A relatively common polymorphism resulting in a substitution of leucine for valine at position 34 (V34L) of the catalytic subunit appears to confer functional changes on FXIII, affecting both its thrombin-induced activation as well as its intrinsic enzymatic activity. To date, controversial data concerning the role of V34L polymorphism of FXIII gene have been reported. An increased risk of sporadic ICH in V34L carriers was reported in two case-control studies [68,69], while another study did not observe significant differences in the prevalence of V34L polymorphism among patients with PICH and subarachnoid hemorrhage as compared to controls [70]. Recently, the FXIII L34 allele was found not to be a risk factor for ICH in a Spanish population [71].

Factor V and Factor II

Over the last years, sparse reports have investigated the role of other polymorphisms that affect clotting factors with relevant effect in the levels or function of the encoded proteins and that could be related to spontaneous ICH. A low prevalence of prothrombotic mutations, such as the R/Q 506 mutation in the factor V gene (FV Leiden) and the G/A transition at position 20210 in the 3'untranslated region of the prothrombin gene (FII), was found in a case-control study conducted on 201 PICH and 201 controls [70]. These findings suggest the hypothesis of a protective role of FV Leiden and prothrombin G20210A mutation in bleeding disorders, such as PICH.

Factor VII

The impact of polymorphisms in the factor VII (FVII) on the risk of PICH has been also investigated. FVII is a vitamin-K dependent inactive protease, which is converted to its active form by contact with tissue factor, and whose physiological effect is the activation of factor X and factor IX. In patients suffering from inherited severe FVII deficiency, PICH is common and occurs usually shortly after birth [72]. A higher risk of PICH was reported amongst carriers of the (-323)Ins allele, which leads to decreased FVII plasma levels [70,71]. By contrast, non-significant differences were found in another case-control study, investigating the role of the (401)G→T polymorphism, associated with elevated plasma FVII levels, and the (-402)G→A polymorphism in the promoter region, related to decreased plasma FVII levels [73].

Platelet-activating Factor

A missense mutation (V279F) in the platelet-activating factor (PAF) acetylhydrolase gene, reported primarily in Asian populations has been found to be associated with PICH in a Japanese study [74].

β1-Tubulin

Recently, a polymorphism (Q43P) in β1-tubulin (TUBB1), a protein specifically expressed in the megakaryocytic line and affecting platelet function, has been linked to PICH in a Spanish case-control study [71]. Interestingly, in this study, a synergist effect was found when TUBB1 Q43P polymorphism was combined with other pro-hemorrhagic polymorphisms, such as FVII –323 Del/Ins and FXIII V34L polymorphisms. Conversely, the pro-thrombotic polymorphism, HPA-1b (GPIIIa L33P), was not found to increase the risk of PICH neither alone nor in combination with TUBB1 Q43P polymorphism [71].

Other Genetic Pathways

The role of other polymorphisms as susceptibility factors in spontaneous ICH has been described in the last years, providing evidence for different genetic contributions to the pathophysiological processes of ICH. Among these, the polymorphism A15T of the SERPINA3 (previously known as α1-antichymotrypsin, ACT) gene, encoding a protease inhibitor that regulates the activity of serine proteases such as neutrophil cathepsin G, has been investigated in several association studies. To date the observations on a possible role of this protease inhibitor in cerebral bleeding are controversial. The TT genotype has been found to be associated with PICH in a Spanish population [75], whereas a Polish study failed to find an association [76]. Although other data sets are requested, the possibility that the ACT-TT genotype might facilitate proteolytic rupture of vessels that harbor amyloidotic changes [75] or might be in linkage disequilibrium with other mutations in this or in other genes cannot be ruled out.

A potential involvement in sporadic ICH has been suggested for a component of the transforming growth factor-beta (TGF-β) receptor complex, the endoglin (ENG), predominantly expressed on the surface of endothelial cells. ENG plays a role in vascular development and remodeling. Impairment of ENG function diminishes the response of the endothelium to TGF-β, resulting in vascular disease. Mutations in this gene are associated with hereditary hemorrhagic telangiectasia (HHT) [77]. A case-control study of 103 patients with PICH and 202 controls showed that carriers of homozygosity for a 6-base insertion in intron 7 of ENG gene was associated with a 4.8-fold increased risk of PICH [78].

Hypertension is the most important risk factor for spontaneous ICH [2], in particular among cases of non-lobar ICH [6]. In spite of this, not every hypertensive individual develops ICH, nor can every case of non-lobar ICH be ascribed to hypertension. Occurrence of an ischemic stroke, ICH or stroke at all is probably influenced by the presence or absence of additional risk factors [79]. Hypertension is, at least partially, genetically determined [80,81]. A recent study of familial clustering of ICH found that 14 out of 144 prospectively assessed PICH patients had a family history of ICH including 9 out of 75 patients with hemorrhage in deep brain structures typical of hypertensive hemorrhage. This suggests a possible involvement of susceptibility genes in this pathological process [11]. However, too few studies have investigated candidate genes specific for hypertensive hemorrhage pathways to date. Similarly, little and conflicting data are available on the relation between ICH and one of the most extensively studied polymorphisms in vascular disease, the insertion/deletion (I/D) in intron 16 of the angiotensin converting enzyme (ACE) gene. While a ACE DD was found to increase the risk for ICH in a Polish population [82], another case-control study looking for the association with I/D polymorphism and its relation with ACE activity in ICH patients showed negative results [83].

Genetics of Vascular Malformations

The most common vascular abnormalities associated with intracerebral bleeding are AVMs and cavernous hemangiomas. There is a tendency for these lesions to run in families. Furthermore, certain rare, well-characterized, familial or congenital syndromes, such as HHT, include cerebrovascular malformations among their constellation of abnormalities. This suggests that a genetic component is at least involved in some secondary causes of ICH, such as hereditary syndromes featuring AVMs and cavernous hemangiomas.

Hereditary Syndrome Featuring AVMs

AVMs are a tangled bundle of malformed blood vessels, specifically, a vascular conglomerate with complex twists, linked by one or more fistulae. An important anatomical feature of this vascular conglomerate, also known as the nidus, is the lack of a capillary bed. Arteries feeding are directly connected to the draining veins (shunting). Most commonly,

AVMs are singular lesions that hemorrhage into the subcortical white matter. Patients with AVMs commonly present with intracranial hemorrhage, which can be primarily parenchymal, subarachnoid, ventricular or any combination of these, according to the site of the lesion and its angioarchitecture [84]. Other common clinical features are seizure, headache and, rarely, evolving focal neurological deficits after ICH. AVMs represent approximately 2% of all ICH with an annual risk of re-hemorrhage approximating 18% [85]. Cerebral AVMs are recognized as part of an inherited disease, HHT, in which a genetic factor has been clearly identified, but also associated with rare congenital syndrome such as Wyburn-Mason syndrome, von Hippel-Lindau disease and Sturge-Weber disease [85]. Apart from these cases, cerebral AVMs are rarely familial.

Hereditary Hemorrhagic Telangiectasia

HHT, also known as Rendu-Osler-Weber syndrome, is an autosomal dominant vascular dysplasia with an estimated incidence of 1/10000 [86] and an almost complete penetrance above the age of 40 years. Characteristic manifestations include epistaxes, telangiectasias, and AVMs. Telangiectasias are small vascular lesions located predominantly on the face, lips, hands, and in oral, nasal and gastrointestinal mucosa. AVMs are larger vascular lesions found in solid organs, most commonly in the lung, liver, and central nervous system. Vascular malformations affecting the brain are primarily AVMs. Symptomatic cerebral AVMs are present in up to 5% of patients with HHT [87,88]. Screening for asymptomatic lesions reveals a higher incidence (nearly 13%) [89,90]. Families with this uncommon angiodysplastic disorder often have multiple cerebral AVMs. Up to one third of HHT patients harboring AVMs have multiple lesions [88,91].

HHT is a genetically and clinically heterogenous disorder. To date, two genes for HHT have been mapped: the ENG gene to the long arm of the chromosome 9 [77], and the activin receptor-like kinase 1 (ALK1) gene to the chromosome 12 q [92], underlying the HHT types 1 and 2, respectively. More than 150 ENG mutations and 120 ALK1 mutations have been reported [86]. Both the ENG and ALK1 proteins are members of the TGF-β family, which is involved in many functions, including vasculogenesis, wound repair and angiogenesis. Endoglin is a receptor for TGF-β, specifically the type III TGF-β receptor, while ALK1 is one of the type I TGF-β receptors. Both these proteins are expressed exclusively on endothelial cells. Although HHT1 and HHT2 highlight the role of receptors for TGF-β family members in vascular differentiation, the pathogenetic mechanism of the TGF-β pathway in these disorders is not clear.

Distinct genotype-phenotype correlations have been observed in HHT, with both intra- and interfamilial variations in age-of-onset, localization of lesions, and severity of complications. It has been suggested that pulmonary AVMs are more common in HHT1 than in HHT2 [93], whereas hepatic AVMs are characteristic of HHT2 [94]. HHT2 also has later onset and lower penetrance [95]. Recently, studies based on the linkage analysis approach detected two other genes underlying HHT located on chromosome 5q (HHT3) [96] and 7p (HHT4) [97].

Cerebral Cavernous Hemangiomas

Cerebral cavernous hemangiomas (or cerebral cavernous malformation, CCM) consist of contiguous endothelial cell lined spaces (caverns) filled with blood or thrombus at various stages of organization, lacking mature vascular wall angioarchitecture, and surrounded by a gliotic margin with uniform features of blood leakage and chronic hemorrhage. CCM can be asymptomatic resulting as incidental findings on neuroimaging. Other possible clinical manifestations (besides ICH) include seizures, progressive neurological signs and headache. The prevalence of CCM has been estimated to be close to 0,1-0,5% in the general population [98]. The annual lesion hemorrhage rate varies from 0.1% to 1.1% per year for the first hemorrhage [98-100] while the annual risk of recurrent hemorrhage is estimated at 4,5%, which can be reduced by surgical intervention [101]. CCM are either sporadic or a familial autosomal dominant condition. Usually, sporadic cases are characterized by a single lesion whereas patients with familial cavernomas have multiple lesions, the number of which is strongly correlated to patient's age [102,103]. The familial form of the disease affects up to 30-50% of patients harboring a CCM [104] and presents with an autosomal dominant pattern of inheritance. At least four loci have been reported to be associated with CCM. CCM1 has been localized on chromosome 7q11-12 with mutations in KRIT 1 (Krev interaction trapped 1) gene [105,106] which encodes a 736-amino acid protein containing four ankyrin domains and a FERM domain. This protein has been shown to interact in vitro with Rap1A, a small Ras-like GTPase, and ICAP-1α, a modulator of β1 integrin signal transduction pathway, as well as with the Ccm2 protein. So far, more than 90 distinct CCM1 mutations have been identified, all of which lead to premature termination codons. This suggests that a loss of function, through mRNA decay of the mutated allele, is the most likely pathophysiological mechanism involved in CCM1 patients.

CCM2 has been found on chromosome 7p13 with MGC4607 or malcaverin mutations [107,108]. The encoded protein contains a phosphotyrosine binding domain similar to that of ICAP-1α and it is able to interact with KRIT1, thus suggesting that ICAP-1α, KRIT1 and CCM2 function in the same signaling pathway. CCM3 has been mapped on chromosome 3q26.1 with mutations in PDCD10 gene [109]. The proportions of families linked to these loci have been estimated to be close to 40% (CCM1), 20% (CCM2), and 40% (CCM3) [110-112]. Recently, a linkage analysis approach allowed to map another locus, CCM4, on chromosome 3q26.3-27.2 [113].

Practical Implications

Genetics of ICH is still in its infancy. Information generated by studies on the genetic aspects of the disease has benefited our understanding of the pathophysiology of ICH, pointing towards specific genes and alleles with roles in the disease process. Like in other complex polygenic diseases, whether genetic information can also routinely benefit clinical practice in this area remains to be determined, but it is plausible that genetic factors might influence clinical decisions such as whether to treat particular individuals with anticoagulants or thrombolytics. Another area in which genetic information is likely to prove useful is in the design and analysis of clinical drug trials for ICH, potentially allowing patients to be stratified according to their predicted clinical course.

References

[1] Dennis MS, Burn JP, Sandercock PA, Bamford JM, Wade DT, Warlow CP. (1993) Long-term survival after first-ever stroke: the Oxfordshire Community Stroke Project. *Stroke*. 24:796-800.

[2] Qureshi AI, Tuhrim S, Broderick JP, Batjer HH, Hondo H, Hanley DF. (2001) Spontaneous intracerebral hemorrhage. *N. Engl. J. Med.* 344:1450-1460.

[3] Broderick J, Brott T, Tomsick T, Huster G. (1993) Intracerebral hemorrhage is more than twice as common as subarachnoid hemorrhage. *J. Neurosurg*. 78:188-191.

[4] Broderick J. Intracerebral hemorrhage. In: Gorelick P, Alter M, eds. (1994) Handbook of Neuroepidemiology. New York: Marcel Dekker Inc. 141-167.

[5] Hill MD, Silver FL, Austin PC, Tu JV. (2000) Rate of stroke recurrence in patients with primary intracerebral hemorrhage. *Stroke*. 31:123-7.

[6] Woo D, Sauerbeck LR, Kissela BM, Khoury JC, Szaflarski JP, Gebel J, Shukla R, Pancioli AM, Jauch EC, Menon AG, Deka R, Carrozzella JA, Moomaw CJ, Fontaine RN, Broderick JP. (2002) Genetic and environmental risk factors for intracerebral hemorrhage. *Stroke*. 33:1190-1195.

[7] Thrift AG, McNeil JJ, Forbes A, Donnan GA. (1998) Three important subgroups of hypertensive persons at greater risk of intracerebral hemorrhage. Melbourne Risk Factor Study Group. *Hypertension*. 31:1223-9.

[8] Hylek EM, Singer DE. (1994) Risk factors for intracranial hemorrhage in outpatients taking warfarin. *Ann. Intern. Med.* 120:897-902

[9] Monforte R, Estruch R, Graus F, Nicolas JM, Urbano-Marquez A. (1990) High ethanol consumption as risk factor for intracerebral hemorrhage in young and middle-aged people. *Stroke*. 21:1529-32.

[10] Ariesen MJ, Claus SP, Rinkel GJE, Algra A. (2003). Risk factors for intracerebral hemorrhage in the general population: a systematic review. *Stroke*. 34:2060-2065.

[11] Alberts MJ, McCarron MO, Hoffmann KL, Graffagnino C. (2002) Familial clustering of intracerebral hemorrhage: a prospective study in North Carolina. *Neuroepidemiology*. 21:18-21.

[12] Polychronopoulos P, Gioldasis G, Ellul J, Metallinos IC, Lekka NP, Paschalis C, Papapetropoulos T. (2002) Family history of stroke in stroke types and subtypes. *J. Neurol. Sci.* 195:117-122.

[13] Bak S, Gaist D, Sindrup SH, Skytthe A, Christensen K. (2002) Genetic liability in stroke: a long-term follow-up study of Danish twins. *Stroke*. 33:769-74.

[14] Hademenos GJ, Alberts MJ, Awad I, Mayberg M, Shepard T, Jagoda A, Latchaw RE, Todd HW, Viste K, Starke R, Girgus MS, Marler J, Emr M, Hart N. (2001) Advances in the genetics of cerebrovascular disease and stroke. *Neurology*. 56:997-1008.

[15] Alberts MJ. (2001) Genetics update: impact of the human genome projects and identification of a stroke gene. *Stroke*. 32:1239-1241.

[16] Itoh Y, Yamada M, Hayakawa M, Otomo E, Miyatake T. (1993) Cerebral amyloid angiopathy: a significant cause of cerebellar as well as lobar cerebral hemorrhage in the elderly. *J. Neurol. Sci.* 116:135-41.

[17] Castano EM, Frangione B. (1988). Human amyloidosis, Alzheimer disease and related disorders. Lab Invest. 58:122-132.

[18] Yamada M. (2000). Cerebral amyloid angiopathy: an overview. *Neuropathology*. 20:8-22.

[19] Revesz T, Ghiso J, Lashley T, Plant G, Rostagno A, Frangione B, Holton JL. (2003) Cerebral amyloid angiopathies: a pathologic, biochemical and genetic view. *J. Neuropathol. Exp. Neurol.* 62:885-98.

[20] Rensink AA, de Waal RM, Kremer B, Verbeek MM. (2003) Pathogenesis of cerebral amyloid angiopathy. *Brain Res. Brain Res. Rev*. 43:2007-223.

[21] Haan J, Maat-Schieman MLC, Roos RAC. (1994) Clinical effects of cerebral amyloid angiopathy. *Dementia*. 5:210-213.

[22] Vinters HV. (1987) Cerebral amyloid angiopathy. A critical review. *Stroke*. 18:311-324.

[23] Greenberg SM. (1998) Cerebral amyloid angiopathy: prospects for clinical diagnosis and treatment. *Neurology*. 51:690-694.

[24] Knudsen KA, Rosand J, Karluk D, Greenberg SM. (2001) Clinical diagnosis of cerebral amyloid angiopathy: validation of the Boston criteria. *Neurology*. 56:537-9.

[25] Vonsattel JP, Myers RH, Hedley-White ET, Ropper AH, Bird ED, Richardson Jr EP. (1991) Cerebral amyloid angiopathy without and with cerebral hemorrhage: a comparative histological study. *Ann. Neurol*. 30:637-649.

[26] Haan J. (2003) Genetics of intracerebral hemorrhage. In Markus H (Ed.), Stroke genetics, Oxford, Oxford University Press, 223-241.

[27] Van Broeckhoven C, Haan J, Bakker E, Hardy JA, Van Hul W, Wehnert A, Vegter-Van der Vlis M, Roos RA. (1990) Amyloid beta protein precursor gene and hereditary cerebral hemorrhage with amyloidosis (Dutch). *Science*. 248:1120-1122.

[28] Miravalle L, Tokuda T, Chiarle R, Giaccone G, Bugiani O, Tagliavini F, Frangione B, Ghiso J. (2000) Substitutions at codon 22 of Alzheimer's Abeta peptide induce diverse conformational changes and apoptotic effects in human cerebral endothelial cells. *J. Biol. Chem.* 275:27110-27116.

[29] Hendriks L, van Duijn CM, Cras P, Cruts M, Van Hul W, van Harskamp F, Warren A, McInnis MG, Antonarakis SE, Martin JJ, et al. (1992) Presenile dementia and cerebral hemorrhage linked to a mutation at codon 692 of the beta-amyloid precursor protein gene. *Nat. Genet.* 1:218-221.

[30] Grabowski TJ, Cho HS, Vonsattel JP, Rebeck GW, Greenberg SM. (2001) Novel amyloid precursor protein mutation in an Iowa family with dementia and severe cerebral amyloid angiopathy. *Ann. Neurol*. 49:697-705.

[31] Cras P, van Harskamp F, Hendriks L, Ceuterick C, van Duijn CM, Stefanko SZ, Hofman A, Kros JM, Van Broeckhoven C, Martin JJ. (1998) Presenile Alzheimer dementia characterized by amyloid angiopathy and large amyloid core type senile plaques in the APP 692Ala→Gly mutation. *Acta. Neuropathol.* (Berl) 96:253-260.

[32] Levy-Lahad E, Wasco W, Poorkaj P, Romano DM, Oshima J, Pettingell WH, Yu CE, Jondro PD, Schmidt SD, Wang K. (1995) Candidate gene for the chromosome 1 familial Alzheimer's disease locus. *Science.* 269:973-977.

[33] Van Dorpe J, Smeijers L, Dewachter I, Nuyens D, Spittaels K, Van Den Haute C, Mercken M, Moechars D, Laenen I, Kuiperi C, Bruynseels K, Tesseur I, Loos R, Vanderstichele H, Checler F, Sciot R, Van Leuven F. (2000) Prominent cerebral amyloid angiopathy in transgenic mice overexpressing the London mutant of human APP in neurons. *Am. J. Pathol.* 157:1283-1298.

[34] Bornebroek M, Haan J, Maat-Schieman ML, Van Duinen SG, Roos RA. (1996) Hereditary cerebral hemorrhage with amyloidosis-Dutch type (HCHWA-D): I. A review of clinical, radiologic and genetic aspects. *Brain Pathol.* 6:111-114.

[35] Davis J, Van Nostrand WE. (1996) Enhanced pathologic properties of Dutch-type mutant amyloid beta-protein. *Proc. Natl. Acad. Sci. USA*. 93:2996-3000.

[36] Melchor JP, McVoy L, Van Nostrand WE. (2000) Charge alterations of E22 enhance the pathogenic properties of the amyloid beta-protein. *J. Neurochem*. 74:2209-12.

[37] Eisenhauer PB, Johnson RJ, Wells JM, Davies TA, Fine RE. (2000) Toxicity of various amyloid beta peptide species in cultured human blood-brain barrier endothelial cells: Increased toxicity of Dutch-type mutant. *J. Neurosci. Res*. 60:804-810.

[38] Wang Z, Natté R, Berliner JA, van Duinen SG, Vinters HV. (2000) Toxicity of Dutch (E22Q) and Flemish (A21G) mutant amyloid beta proteins to human cerebral microvessel and aortic smooth muscle cells. *Stroke.* 31:534-538.

[39] Van Nostrand WE, Melchor JP, Cho HS, Greenberg SM, Rebeck GW. (2001) Pathogenic Effects of D23N Iowa Mutant Amyloid beta-Protein. *J. Biol. Chem.* 276:32860-32866.

[40] Selkoe DJ. (1999) Translating cell biology into therapeutic advances in Alzheimer's disease. *Nature*. 399(6738 Suppl):A23-31.

[41] De Jonghe C, Zehr C, Yager D, Prada CM, Younkin S, Hendriks L, Van Broeckhoven C, Eckman CB. (1998) Flemish and Dutch mutations in amyloid beta precursor protein have different effects on amyloid beta secretion. *Neurobiol. Dis*. 5:281-286.

[42] Levy E, Lopez-Otin C, Ghiso J, Geltner D, Frangione B. (1989) Stroke in Icelandic patients with hereditary amyloid angiopathy is related to a mutation in the cystatin C gene, an inhibitor of cysteine proteases. *J. Exp. Med.* 169:1771-8.

[43] Vidal R, Frangione B, Rostagno A, Mead S, Révész T, Plant G, Ghiso J. (1999) A stop-codon mutation in the BRI gene associated with familial British dementia. *Nature.* 399:776-81.

[44] Mead S, James-Galton M, Revesz T, Doshi RB, Harwood G, Pan EL, Ghiso J, Frangione B, Plant G. (2000) Familial British dementia with amyloid angiopathy: early clinical, neuropsychological and imaging findings. *Brain.* 123:975-91.

[45] Nochlin D, Bird TD, Nemens EJ, Ball MJ, Sumi SM. (1998) Amyloid angiopathy in a Volga German family with Alzheimer's disease and a presenilin-2 mutation (N141I). *Ann. Neurol.* 43:131-5.

[46] Sánchez-Valle R, Lladó A, Ezquerra M, Rey MJ, Rami L, Molinuevo JL. (2007) A novel mutation in the PSEN1 gene (L286P) associated with familial early-onset dementia of Alzheimer type and lobar haematomas. *Eur. J. Neurol.* 14:1409-12.

[47] Graffagnino C, Herbstreith MH, Roses AD, Alberts MJ. (1994) A molecular genetic study of intracerebral hemorrhage. *Arch. Neurol.* 51:981-4.

[48] Graffagnino C, Herbstreith MH, Schmechel DE, Levy E, Roses AD, Alberts MJ. (1995) Cystatin C mutation in an elderly man with sporadic amyloid angiopathy and intracerebral hemorrhage. *Stroke.* 26:2190-2193.

[49] McCarron MO, Nicoll JA, Stewart J, et al: (2000) Absence of cystatin C mutation in sporadic cerebral amyloid angiopathy-related hemorrhage. *Neurology.* 54:242-244.

[50] McCarron MO, Nicoll JA, Ironside JW, Love S, Alberts MJ, Bone I. (1999) Cerebral amyloid angiopathy-related hemorrhage. Interaction of APOE ε2 with putative clinical risk factors. *Stroke.* 30:1643-6.

[51] Greenberg SM, Briggs ME, Hyman BT, Kokoris GJ, Takis C, Kanter DS, Kase CS, Pessin MS. (1996) Apolipoprotein E epsilon 4 is associated with the presence and earlier onset of hemorrhage in cerebral amyloid angiopathy. *Stroke.* 27:1333-7.

[52] O'Donnell HC, Rosand J, Knudsen KA, Furie KL, Segal AZ, Chiu RI, Ikeda D, Greenberg SM. (2000) Apolipoprotein E genotype and the risk of recurrent lobar intracerebral hemorrhage. *N. Engl. J. Med.* 342:240-245.

[53] Premkumar DR, Cohen DL, Hedera P, Friedland RP, Kalaria RN. (1996) Apolipoprotein E-epsilon4 alleles in cerebral amyloid angiopathy and cerebrovascular pathology associated with Alzheimer's disease. *Am. J. Pathol.* 148:2083-2095.

[54] Greenberg SM, Rebeck GW, Vonsattel JPG, Gomes-Isla T, Hyman BT. (1995) Apolipoprotein E ε4 and cerebral hemorrhage associated with amyloid angiopathy. *Ann. Neurol.* 38:254-259.

[55] Nicoll JA, Burnett C, Love S, Graham DI, Dewar D, Ironside JW, Stewart J, Vinters HV. (1997) High frequency of apolipoprotein ε2 allele in hemorrhage due to cerebral amyloid angiopathy. *Ann. Neurol.* 41:716-721.

[56] McCarron MO, Nicoll JA. (1998) High frequency of apolipoprotein E ε2 allele is specific for patients with cerebral amyloid angiopathy related-hemorrhage. *Neurosci. Lett.* 247:45-48.

[57] Yamada M, Itoh Y, Suematsu N, Matsushita M, Otomo E. (1996) Lack of an association between apolipoprotein E ε4 and cerebral amyloid angiopathy in elderly Japanese. *Ann. Neurol.* 39:683-684.

[58] Sudlow C, Martínez González NA, Kim J, Clark C. (2006) Does apolipoprotein E genotype influence the risk of ischemic stroke, intracerebral hemorrhage, or subarachnoid hemorrhage? Systematic review and meta-analyses of 31 studies among 5961 cases and 17,965 controls. *Stroke.* 37:364-70.

[59] McCarron MO, Nicoll JA. (2000a) Apolipoprotein E genotype and cerebral amyloid angiopathy-related hemorrhage. *Ann. N. Y. Acad. Sci.* 903:961-965.

[60] del Zoppo GJ, Mori E. (1992) Hematologic causes of intracerebral hemorrhage and their treatment. *Neurosurg Clin N Am.* 3:637-58.

[61] Gebel JM, Broderick JP. (2000) Intracerebral hemorrhage. *Neurol. Clin.* 18:419-38.

[62] Zodpey SP, Tiwari RR, Kulkarni HR. (2000) Risk factors for haemorrhagic stroke: a case-control study. *Public Health.* 114:177-82.

[63] Hart RG, Boop BS, Anderson DC. (1995) Oral anticoagulants and intracranial hemorrhage. Facts and hypotheses. *Stroke.* 26:1471-7.

[64] Gorter JW. (1999) Major bleeding during anticoagulation after cerebral ischemia: patterns and risk factors. Stroke Prevention In Reversible Ischemia Trial (SPIRIT). European Atrial Fibrillation Trial (EAFT) study groups. *Neurology*. 53:1319-27.

[65] Rosand J, Hylek EM, O'Donnell HC, Greenberg SM. (2000) Warfarin-associated hemorrhage and cerebral amyloid angiopathy: a genetic and pathologic study. *Neurology*. 55:947-51.

[66] Ortel TL. (1999).Genetics of coagulation disorders. In: Genetics of cerebrovascular disease. MJ Alberts (Ed). Futura Publishing Company, New York. 129-156.

[67] Prengler M, Pavlakis SG, Prohovnik I, Adams RJ. (2002) Sickle cell disease: the neurological complications. *Ann. Neurol.* 51:543-52.

[68] Catto AJ, Kohler HP, Bannan S, Stickland M, Carter A, Grant PJ. (1998) Factor XIII Val 34 Leu: a novel association with primary intracerebral hemorrhage. *Stroke*. 29:813-6.

[69] Gemmati D, Serino ML, Ongaro A, Tognazzo S, Moratelli S, Resca R, Moretti M, Scapoli GL. (2001) A common mutation in the gene for coagulation factor XIII-A (VAL34Leu): a risk factor for primary intracerebral hemorrhage is protective against atherothrombotic diseases. *Am. J. Hematol.* 67:183-8.

[70] Corral J, Iniesta JA, González-Conejero R, Villalón M, Rivera J, Vicente V. (2000) Factor XIII Val34Leu polymorphism in primary intracerebral haemorrhage. *Hematol. J.* 1:269-73.

[71] Navarro-Núñez L, Lozano ML, Rivera J, Corral J, Roldán V, González-Conejero R, Iniesta JA, Montaner J, Vicente V, Martínez C. (2007) The association of the beta1-tubulin Q43P polymorphism with intracerebral hemorrhage in men. *Haematologica.* 92:513-8.

[72] Perry DJ. (2002) Factor VII deficiency. *Br. J. Haematol.* 118:689-700.

[73] Greisenegger S, Weber M, Funk M, Endler G, Lang W, Ferrari J, Lalouschek W. (2007) Polymorphisms in the coagulation factor VII gene and risk of primary intracerebral hemorrhage. *Eur. J. Neurol.* 14:1098-1101.

[74] Yoshida H, Imaizumi T, Fujimoto K, Itaya H, Hiramoto M, Yoshimizu N, Fukushi K, Satoh K. (1998) A mutation in plasma platelet-activating factor acetylhydrolase (Val279Phe) is a genetic risk factor for cerebral hemorrhage but not for hypertension. *Thromb Haemost*. 80:372-375.

[75] Obach V, Revilla M, Vila N, Cervera A A, Chamorro A A. (2001) alpha(1)-antichymotrypsin polymorphism: a risk factor for hemorrhagic stroke in normotensive subjects. *Stroke*. 32:2588-91.

[76] Pera J, Slowik A, Dziedzic T, Szczudlik A. (2006) SERPINA3 polymorphism is not associated with primary intracerebral hemorrhage in a Polish population. *Stroke.* 37:906-907.

[77] McAllister KA, Grogg KM, Johnson DW, Gallione CJ, Baldwin MA, Jackson CE, Helmbold EA, Markel DS, McKinnon WC, Murrell J, et al. (1994) Endoglin, a TGF-beta binding protein of endothelial cells, is the gene for hereditary haemorrhagic telangiectasia type 1. *Nat. Genet.* 8:345-51.

[78] Alberts MJ, Davis JP, Graffagnino C, McClenny C, Delong D, Granger C, Herbstreith MH, Boteva K, Marchuk DA, Roses AD. (1997) Endoglin gene polymorphism as a risk factor for sporadic intracerebral hemorrhage. *Ann. Neurol.* 41:683-6.

[79] Bogousslavsky J, Castillo V, Kumral E, Henriques I, Melle GV. (1996) Stroke subtypes and hypertension. Primary hemorrhage vs infarction, large- vs small-artery disease. *Arch. Neurol.* 53:265-269.

[80] Svetkey LP, O'Riordan E, Conlon PJ, Emovon O. (1999) Genetics of hypertension. In: Genetics of cerebrovascular disease. Alberts MJ (Ed). Futura Publishing Company, New York. 57-80.

[81] Doris PA. (2002) Hypertension genetics, single nucleotide polymorphisms, and the common disease: common variant hypothesis. *Hypertension.* 39:323-31.

[82] Slowik A, Turaj W, Dziedzic T, Haefele A, Pera J, Malecki MT, Glodzik-Sobanska L, Szermer P, Figlewicz DA, Szczudlik A. (2004) DD genotype of ACE gene is a risk factor for intracerebral hemorrhage. *Neurology.* 63:359-361.

[83] Catto A, Carter AM, Barrett JH, Stickland M, Bamford J, Davies JA, Grant PJ. (1996) Angiotensin-converting enzyme insertion/deletion polymorphism and cerebrovascular disease. *Stroke.* 27:435-40.

[84] Choi JH, Mohr JP. (2005) Brain arteriovenous malformations in adults. *Lancet Neurol.* 4:299-308.

[85] Arteriovenous malformations of the brain in adults. (1999) *N. Engl. J. Med.* 340:1812-8

[86] Abdalla SA, Letarte M. (2006) Hereditary haemorrhagic telangiectasia: current views on genetics and mechanisms of disease. *J. Med. Genet.* 43:97-110.

[87] Guttmacher AE, Marchuk DA, White RI Jr. (1995) Hereditary hemorrhagic telangiectasia. *N. Engl. J. Med.* 333:918-924.

[88] Maher CO, Piepgras DG, Brown RD Jr, Friedman JA, Pollock BE. (2001) Cerebrovascular manifestations in 321 cases of hereditary hemorrhagic telangiectasia. *Stroke.* 32:877-882.

[89] Haitjema T, Disch F, Overtoom TT, Westermann CJ, Lammers JW. (1995) Screening family members of patients with hereditary hemorrhagic telangiectasia. *Am. J. Med.* 99:519-524.

[90] Willemse RB, Mager JJ, Westermann CJ, Overtoom TT, Mauser H, Wolbers JG. (2000) Bleeding risk of cerebrovascular malformations in hereditary hemorrhagic telangiectasia. *J. Neurosurg.* 92:779-784.

[91] Putman CM, Chaloupka JC, Fulbright RK, Awad IA, White RI Jr, Fayad PB. (1996) Exceptional multiplicity of cerebral arteriovenous malformations associated with hereditary hemorrhagic telangiectasia (Osler-Weber-Rendu syndrome). *AJNR Am. J. Neuroradiol.* 17:1733-1742.

[92] Johnson DW, Berg JN, Baldwin MA, Gallione CJ, Marondel I, Yoon SJ, Stenzel TT, Speer M, Pericak-Vance MA, Diamond A, Guttmacher AE, Jackson CE, Attisano L, Kucherlapati R, Porteous ME, Marchuk DA. (1996) Mutations in the activin receptor like kinase 1 gene in hereditary haemorrhagic telangiectasia type 2. *Nat. Genet.* 13:189-195.

[93] Berg JN, Guttmacher AE, Marchuk DA, Porteous ME. (1996) Clinical heterogeneity in hereditary haemorrhagic telangiectasia: Are pulmonary arteriovenous malformations more common in families linked to endoglin? *J. Med. Genet.* 33:256–257.

[94] Olivieri C, Mira E, Delu G, Pagella F, Zambelli A, Malvezzi L, Buscarini E, Danesino C. (2002) Identification of 13 new mutations in the ACVRL1 gene in a group of 52 unselected Italian patients affected by hereditary haemorrhagic telangiectasia. *J. Med. Genet.* 39:e39.

[95] Berg J, Porteous M, Reinhardt D, Gallione C, Holloway S, Umasunthar T, Lux A, McKinnon W, Marchuk D, Guttmacher A. (2003) Hereditary haemorrhagic telangiectasia: A questionnaire based study to delineate the different phenotypes caused by endoglin and ALK1 mutations. *J. Med. Genet.* 40:585–590.

[96] Cole SG, Begbie ME, Wallace GM, Shovlin CL. (2005) A new locus for hereditary haemorrhagic telangiectasia (HHT3) maps to chromosome 5. J Med Genet. 42:577-82

[97] Bayrak-Toydemir P, McDonald J, Akarsu N, Toydemir RM, Calderon F, Tuncali T, Tang W, Miller F, Mao R. (2006) A fourth locus for hereditary hemorrhagic telangiectasia maps to chromosome 7. *Am. J. Med. Genet.* 140:2155-62.

[98] Robinson JR, AwadIA, Little JR. (1991) Natural history of the cavernous angiomas. *J. Neurosurg.* 75:709-714.

[99] Zabramski JM, Wascher TM, Spetzler RF, Johnson B, Golfinos J, Drayer BP, Brown B, Rigamonti D, Brown G. (1994). The natural history of familial cavernous malformations: results of an ongoing study. *J. Neurosurg.* 80:422-432.

[100] Porter PJ, Willinsky RA, Harper W, Wallace MC. (1997) Cerebral cavernous malformations: Natural history and prognosis after clinical deterioration with or without hemorrhage. *J. Neurosurg.* 87:190-197.

[101] Badjatia N, Rosand J. (2005) Intracerebral hemorrhage. *Neurologist.* 11:311-24.

[102] Denier C, Labauge P, Bergametti F, Marchelli F, Riant F, Arnoult M, Maciazek J, Vicaut E, Brunereau L, Tournier-Lasserve E and Société Francaise de Neurochirurgie. (2006). Genotype-phenotype correlations in cerebral cavernous malformations patients. *Ann. Neurol.* 60:550-556.

[103] Labauge P, Laberge S, Brunereau L, Levy C, Tournier-Lasserve E and Société Francaise de Neurochirurgie. (1998) Hereditary cerebral cavernous angiomas: clinical and genetic features in 57 French families. *Lancet.* 352:1892-1897.

[104] Rigamonti D, Hadley MN, Drayer BP, Johnson PC, Hoenig-Rigamonti K, Knight JT, Spetzler RF. (1988) Cerebral cavernous malformations. Incidence and familial occurrence. *N. Engl. J. Med.* 319:343-347.

[105] Laberge-le Couteulx S, Jumg HH, Labauge P, Houtteville JP, Lescoat C, Cecillon M, Marechal E, Joutel A, Bach JF, Tournier-Lasserve E. (1999). Truncating mutations in CCM1, encoding KRIT1, cause cerebral cavernous angiomas. *Nat Genet.* 23:189-193.

[106] Sahoo T, Johnson EW, Thomas JW, Kuehl PM, Jones TL, Dokken CG, Touchman JW, Gallione CJ, Lee-Lin SQ, Kosofsky B, Kurth JH, Louis DN, Mettler G, Morrison L, Gil-Nagel A, Rich SS, Zabramski JM, Boguski MS, Green ED, Marchuk DA. (1999) Mutations in the gene encoding KRIT1, a Krev-1/rap1a binding protein, cause cerebral cavernous malformations (CCM1). *Hum. Mol. Genet.* 8:2325-2333.

[107] Denier C, Goutagny S, Labauge P, Krivosic V, Arnoult M, Cousin A, Benabid AL, Comoy J, Frerebeau P, Gilbert B, Houtteville JP, Jan M, Lapierre F, Loiseau H, Menei P, Mercier P, Moreau JJ, Nivelon-Chevallier A, Parker F, Redondo AM, Scarabin JM, Tremoulet M, Zerah M, Maciazek J, Tournier-Lasserve E; Société Française de Neurochirurgie. (2004) Mutations within the MGC4607 gene cause cerebral cavernous malformations. *Am. J. Hum. Genet.* 74:326-337.

[108] Liquori CL, Berg MJ, Siegel AM, Huang E, Zawistowski JS, Stoffer T, Verlaan D, Balogun F, Hughes L, Leedom TP, Plummer NW, Cannella M, Maglione V, Squitieri F, Johnson EW, Rouleau GA, Ptacek L, Marchuk DA. (2003) Mutations in a gene encoding a novel protein containing a phosphotyrosine-binding domain cause type 2 cerebral cavernous malformations. *Am. J. Hum. Genet.* 73:1459-1464.

[109] Bergametti F, Denier C, Labauge P, Arnoult M, Boetto S, Clanet M, Coubes P, Echenne B, Ibrahim R, Irthum B, Jacquet G, Lonjon M, Moreau JJ, Neau JP, Parker F, Tremoulet M, Tournier-Lasserve E; Société Française de Neurochirurgie. (2005) Mutations within the programmed cell death 10 gene cause cerebral cavernous malformations. *Am. J. Hum. Genet.* 76:42-51.

[110] Gunel M, Awad IA, Finberg K, Anson JA, Steinberg GK, Batjer HH, Kopitnik TA, Morrison L, Giannotta SL, Nelson-Williams C. (1996) A founder mutation as a cause of cerebral cavernous malformations in Hispanic-Americans. *N. Engl. J. Med.* 334:946-951.

[111] Dubovsky J, Zabramski JM, Kurth J, Spetzler RF, Rich SS, Orr HT, Weber JL. (1995) A gene responsible for cavernou.s malformations of the brain maps to chromosome 7q. *Hum. Mol. Genet.* 4:453-458.

[112] Craig HD, Günel M, Cepeda O, Johnson EW, Ptacek L, Steinberg GK, Ogilvy CS, Berg MJ, Crawford SC, Scott RM, Steichen-Gersdorf E, Sabroe R, Kennedy CT, Mettler G, Beis MJ, Fryer A, Awad IA, Lifton RP. (1998) Multilocus linkage identifies two new loci for a Mendelian form of stroke, cerebral cavernous malformation, at 7p15–13 and 3q25.2-27. *Hum. Mol. Genet.* 7:1851–1858.

[113] Liquori CL, Berg MJ, Squitieri F, Ottenbacher M, Sorlie M, Leedom TP, Cannella M, Maglione V, Ptacek L, Johnson EW, Marchuk DA. (2006). Low frequency of PDCD10 mutations in a panel of CCM3 probands: potential for a fourth CCM locus. *Hum. Mutat.* 27:118.

In: Hypertension, Heredity and Stroke
Editor: Cristina Moratinos and Bruno Cardenas
ISBN 978-1-60741-496-4

Chapter 2

Primary Arterial Hypertension in Obese Children as a Risk Factor of the Development of Premature Atherosclerosis

Maria Hanna Kniażewska and Anna Karolina Obuchowicz
Department of Pediatrics in Bytom, Medical University of Silesia, Katowice, Poland

Abstract

Primary arterial hypertension (HT) in children occurs significantly more often than once assumed. It is the main form of HT in children over 12 years old and is prevalent in the obese. It has been proved that birth weight influences the blood pressure development during the developmental age. According to recent data the percentage of overweight and obese children is rising drastically. It has been proved that the weight gain is accompanied by the increase in blood pressure (1 mmHg per each kilogram gained). Impaired glucose tolerance, disturbances of lipid metabolism, increase in cardiac output, sympathetic and rennin-angiotensin-aldosterone systems' activation, sodium and water retention are caused by excessive development of fatty tissue (especially visceral fat), and these factors support development of HT and early atheromatous lesions. Autopsy studies of children and young individuals in the Bogalusa Heart Study provided important information. Strict dependence between weight gain, systolic pressure, lipid disturbances, smoking and progression of atheromatous changes in the aorta and coronary arteries has been proven. These studies indicate occurrence of atherosclerosis in children and the young with risk factors predisposing to the development of atherosclerosis. Identification of CVD risk factors, constituting the metabolic syndrome (HT and obesity are integral parts of this syndrome) in children, is a subject of numerous currently performed researches. In the recent years researches have shown that adipocytes display significant endocrine and paracrine activity. Biologically active substances (influencing blood pressure regulation) secreted by these cells include among others: leptin, adiponectin, Agouti protein, visfatin, resistin, as well as TGF-β, TNF-α, PAI-1, angiotensinogen, rennin, convertase of the angiotensin, chimase, DIG catepsine, prostaglandin, IGF-1, VEGF, MIF, IL-6, sex hormones (testosterone, estradiol, estrone), glicocortycosteroids. Damage of arterial endothelium and oxidative modification of LDL molecules initiate the atheromatous process. Long-term increase in blood pressure is associated with mechanical injuries of the endothelium. The so-called shear stress, resulting from blood flow, leads to secondary activation of inflammatory process intensifying the atheromatosis. Diagnostics of HT causes in obese children with consideration of factors supporting the development of atherosclerosis (standard HT diagnostics, diagnostic of blood vessel conditions – IMT and vessel vasodilatation capability, evaluation of lipid metabolism and the level of glucose utilization and plasma antioxidant capability, evaluation of the so-called new CVD risk factors – levels of homocysteine, CRP, prothrombotic factors) is currently of great significance in primary CVD prophylaxis. Pharmacotherapy, but most importantly non-pharmacological methods of treatment aiming to modify the lifestyle (weight loss, increase in physical activity, dietary conduct, quitting smoking) are of specific significance in obese children suffering from HT.

Introduction

Despite continuous attempts by the medical profession in many countries, the cardiovascular disease (CVD) is still a main cause of death in both developed and developing countries, killing approximately four million Europeans a year, and is considered to be "the murderer of the 21st century". There is currently no doubt that factors accelerating atherosclerosis include obesity, arterial hypertension, lipid metabolism disorders and impaired glucose tolerance. Among these factors obesity plays a special role, favouring increases of arterial blood pressure, lipid and carbohydrate metabolism disorders, progression of non-alcoholic fatty liver disease, obstructive sleep apnoea, orthopaedic problems and – and this should not be omitted – socioeconomic and emotional problems resulting from low self-esteem [1]. As a result of obesity, not only is there a higher risk of cardiovascular system diseases and diabetes, but also an increased threat from neoplastic disease [2, 3, 4].

The number of obese people in the last 20 years has grown constantly up to the current pandemic levels. According to WHO reports [5], one billion adults in the world are overweight, among which 300 million are obese. More and more often, young people of developmental ages are also suffering. It is reckoned that approximately 17.6 million children under the age of 5 are obese and this number is constantly growing. According to the WHO, since 1980 the number of obese children in the USA has doubled, and obese teenagers tripled [5]. The percentage of overweight and obese young people in European countries varies by region, but in the 13 year old population it oscillates between 3% and 34 %, and in 15 year olds from 5% to 28%, with the majority being male [6]. It has been estimated that European countries are home to about 22 million overweight children (5 million of those obese) [7]. There are regions where obesity among children and teenagers is even more frequent. For example, child obesity in the United Arab Emirates is 2 to 3 times more than in world statistics [8]. It should also be mentioned that obesity and overweightness is being diagnosed in increasingly younger children. Nelson et al. [9] found that 40% of New York children age 2 to 4 years had weight of above 85 percentiles. Similar observations came from the Bogalusa Heart Study [10]. According to recent multi-centre population studies in a group of Polish children age 7 to 9, overweightness was present in 15.8% of the boys and 15% of the girls, with obesity in 3.6% of the boys and 3.7% of the girls [11].

The authors of a report published in 2008 in the International Journal of Obesity, based on a forecasting analysis, stated that by 2030 the number of overweight and obese people will increase to 3.3 billion (57.8% of the world's population) [12]. This increase supposedly refers especially to developing countries that see societal age structuring (aging of societies), wealth increases, changes of life style from limitations on physical activity and changes in the quality and amount of food consumed [12].

Arterial hypertension (HT) occurs in overweight people 6 times more often than in those with correct body mass [13]. Currently, it is estimated that over one billion people in the world have increased blood pressure (BP) values, which indirectly causes 7.1 million deaths a year [14,15]. It has been noticed that systolic pressure of 20 mmHg and diastolic pressure of 10 mmHg above desirable values (115/75 mmHg) are related to a doubling in the risk of mortality due to ischemic heart disease or stroke [14].

In recent years though, opinions on HT pathogenesis in children have changed. While in small children (under 10), kidney diseases were thought to dominate among the reasons for HT, it was found that the participation of primary HT has grown considerably in the older group of children. Due to the difficulty of precise evaluation of correct BP value ranges in the developmental age population (BP values are dependent on age, sex, height, ethnicity and the devices used to measure it), evaluation of the spread of HT in children is not precise enough. It is also known that population studies aimed at wide-spread HT evaluation (especially in this age group) have to consider several BP measurements, which for this type of testing is an additional difficulty. When Sorof et al. [16] tested pressure values in teenagers aged 10 to 19, they repeated the BP measurement three times at various intervals, and reduced the number of those diagnosed with HT from 19% to 9.5 % to 4.5 %. It may therefore be considered that evaluation based on one BP measurement may be overstated by as much as four times. Currently, it is accepted that the frequency of HT occurrence in populations under 18 years of age is from 1 to 5% [16,17,18]. Due to the considerable probability of secondary HT, especially in small children and in children with severe HT, much emphasis is put on thorough diagnostics of the causes. Among the reasons for HT in teenagers, primary HT is dominant, being especially present in relation to obesity, family history of HT and sedentary lifestyle [16]. The cause-and-effect relationship of HT with obesity has been documented sufficiently with numerous studies on adult populations, but also less numerous but equally convincing are the studies in child/teenage groups. Results of studies conducted by Rosner et al. [19] among 47,000 children prove that independently of race, sex and age, arterial blood pressure values increase with BMI centiles. Based on a long-term, wide-ranging population study, the Bogalusa Heart Study on overweight and obese children found systolic high pressure values 4.5 times more frequently and diastolic pressure 2.4 times more frequently, than in their correctly weighted peers [20]. When testing almost 2,500 teenagers, Sorof et al. [21] found that HT is present more frequently in obese people and refers mainly to systolic pressure.

Diagnosis of Obesity and Arterial Hypertension in Children

The somatic development of a person in developmental ages is evaluated by comparing the measurement results of the somatic features of a child with a biological reference system, i.e. appropriate norms. Until recently, the evaluation of correctness of somatic development was made only based on reference between weight and height values with appropriate centile charts or numerical tables. In the last two decades though, it was decided to qualify nutritional disorders in children and teenagers based on a BMI evaluation (*Body Mass Index* - ratios derived by dividing weight in kilograms by height in meters, in a square). Ranges for BMI standards are specified for age, sex, ethnicity and place of residence (geographic regions, urban conurbations, the countryside). However, construction of growth centiles and tables based on population studies has raised certain doubts about the increasing presence of nutritional disorders in children and teenagers which may influence the range of norms established from those studies. According to the majority of authors, obesity is defined based on a BMI exceeding or equal to a value of 95 centiles for age and sex, while overweight is defined by a BMI between 90 and 95 centiles. For individual stratification of entire cardio-vascular risk and for the needs of scientific studies, more precise quantitative and fat tissue distribution evaluation methods are indispensable, and so anthropometric methods are used for this – abdomen circumference measurement, fat folds and calculations based on waist-hip and waist- height ratios. More precise methods include fat tissue content evaluation using the bioelectrical impedance method and distribution evaluation and fat tissue evals using dual-energy X-ray absorptiometry (*DXA*), dual-energy photon absorptiometry, magnetic resonance, computer tomography, isotope dilution techniques, ^{40}K (potassium isotope) total content evaluation and neutron activation analysis – for total calcium and nitrogen content. For that purpose, the easiest and cheapest methods used are Bioelectrical Impedance Analysis (BIA) and DXA [22]. The BIA technique is non-invasive, using the body's own electric properties and the different resistances of different tissues to electric current. This method consists of measuring various tissues' electric resistance to low intensity current, and is used for tissue volume, shape, electric properties' measurement and also for evaluation of total body water, fat and other tissues (fat-free body mass). Dual-energy X-ray absorptiometry is also used to evaluate body composition, including total mineral density, fat-free body mass and fat tissue percentages.

BP measurement in children requires apparatus for BP measurement (often calibrated) with cuffs of various widths adjusted to the child's arm's dimensions. BP measurement values refer to centile charts prepared separately for boys and girls. More precise evaluations are done with consideration to the child's growth centile and by referring to BP values not only to sex and age standards but also the child's height, and this is of significance in interpretation of BP measurement in the very tall or very short. To diagnose HT, systolic and/or diastolic BP values are required which are equal to or higher than 95 centiles for sex, age, and height on at least 3 occasions, performed under standard conditions during several visits to the doctor. Pre-hypertensive state or so-called high-normal BP is defined by BP $\geq$ 90, but < 95 centile values, or as with adults, ≥ 120/80 and ≤ 139/89 [23, 24]. Ambulatory Blood Pressure Monitoring (ABPM) services are invaluable here since they allow not only evaluation in the HT arena but also twenty-four-hour BP rhythm, and can more precisely assess total cardiovascular risk [25, 26]. Nowadays, ABPM is considered a recommended and recognised BP measurement method in children and teens [25,26], however any recommendations regarding ABPM interpretation in this age group are based only on experts' opinions and not on perspective studies evaluating so-called "hard endpoints" (myocardial infarction, stroke) [27]. Certainly, long-tem prospective studies would allow final definition of standard BP values for the developmental age population.

The Course of Arterial Hypertension Pathogenesis in Obesity

From the time of the publishing of the classic American study by Framingham, the pathogenic relationship between arterial hypertension and obesity has been commonly recognised, but the cause of arterial blood pressure increases in obese people has not yet been fully explained [28].

Undoubtedly, activation of sympathetic system participates in generations of higher BP values in those people is proved by an increase of Systolic BP (SBP) and higher heart rate most of all. Among the postulated factors hyperinsulinism, renin-angiotensin-aldosterone system increased activity, increasing volemia of sodium and water retention, and the effect of biologically active substances excreted by fat tissue (hormones and adipocytokines) are also cited.

Special significance is credited to fat tissue distribution which is regulated by hormonal and genetic factors, modified by environmental conditions. In women, fat tissue collects around the hips and subcutaneously, and in men around the abdominal part of the body as a visceral and subcutaneous fat tissue. It is currently known, that an abdominal overweight type enables the presence of both arterial hypertension and metabolic complications. Visceral fat tissue seems to be more metabolically active. The metabolically disadvantageous effect of visceral fat tissue results from, amongst other things, provision of free fat acids via the portal vein to the liver. This intensifies liver cholesterol production, impairs glucose metabolism, decreases cell sensitivity to insulin, and leads to glucose tolerance disorder [29, 30, 31]. Japanese authors, when studying a group of obese children 6 -15 years old found that the SBP level is directly proportional to the degree of visceral obesity, insulin and leptin levels, independently of family history of HT [32]. According to Maffeis et al. [33] abdomen circumference in obese children significantly better correlates with systolic and diastolic (DBP) arterial pressure values than other anthropometric measurements (weight, BMI, skin-fat fold thickness). The authors also showed a statistically strong relationship between this anthropometric parameter and values of some lipid metabolism indexes. Studies conducted in recent years on large patient populations are not definitely clear any more, with regards to the significance of the diversity of fat tissue distribution. Fox et al. [34] published study results conducted within the Framingham Heart Study, where they proved that although the relationship between metabolic risk and visceral fat tissue thickness is very strong, subcutaneous fat tissue amounts also have an effect on every element of this risk (insulin resistance, dyslipidemia, arterial hypertension).

The Role of the Autonomous Nervous System in HT Development in Obese Patients

The coexistence of obesity with hypertension is of a special *perpetuum mobile*. The dependence of BP values on obesity levels has been established, as well as the observation that higher BP increases the risk of obesity [35]. This is related to sympathetic system activation in obese people, which manifests itself by heart action accelerated and BP oscillation. A laboratory proof for sympathetic activation in obese patients is higher catecholamine levels in their blood. Excessive adrenergic system activation in obese people is an effect of many factors including baroreceptor reaction impairment, hypothalamus-pituitary gland axis dysfunction, hyperinsulinism and insulin resistance, hyperleptinemia, renin-angiotensin-aldosterone system activation and obstructive sleep apnoea [36]. It was found that in obese children, resting heart action is quicker than in their slim peers, and is also characterised by higher diversity, which may indirectly indicate sympathetic system activation [21, 37]. A result of long-term intense sympathetic system activity may be decreased sensitivity of β-adrenergic receptors causing difficult elimination of calorific excess delivered with nutrition and weight gain.

In animal studies, special attention has been paid to increased cardiac output in obese individuals, resulting from sympathetic system activation and increased volemia (the result of sodium and water retention), and as a consequence, increases in arterial pressure values. Also, the natriuresis curve dislocation in the direction of higher BP values was also found, which is related to increased tubular sodium reabsorption (an effect of sympathetic system activity increases, the renin-angiotensin-aldosterone system (RAAS), intrarenal pressure increase and hyperinsulinemia) [38].

The RAAS System in Obese and HT Patients

Arterial hypertension in obese patients may have a cause and effect relationship with higher angiotensin II and aldosterone in plasma concentrations. Fat tissue is a source of many of the RAAS system's components which favour BP increases [39]. Causes of higher aldosterone levels in obese people, especially the visceral, is unclear, even more so as aldosterone concentration seems to be independent of plasma rennin activity and potassium levels [40]. Angiotensin II and aldosterone increase volemia by increasing sodium reabsorption in the nephron's proximal tubule, while the angiotensin II also directly causes angiostenosis action in the resistant arteriole by increasing circumferential resistance. Collection of visceral fat tissue around the kidneys and their hilus causes a hydrostatic pressure increase in the kidney itself of 35-40 mmHg, causing this circumferential resistance as well as sodium and water retention [41]. Increased aminoglycan and hyaluronan content in obesity in renal medulla interstitium, additionally causes an increase of intracapsular pressure in the kidneys, as well as Henle's Loop and straight vessels pressure, leading to additional activation of the RAAS system and increased tubular sodium reabsorption [42].

The Role of Hyperinsulinism and Insulin Resistance in HT Development

Studies by many authors have shown an insulin resistance relationship with HT in obese patients. The Bogalusa Heart Study [43] proved the relationship between fasting insulin concentrations and BMI, with BP values in 5 year old children. However, not all studies confirm insulin resistance's role as a causal factor of HT. It is currently known however, that in many people, despite the presence of insulin resistance, BP values remain unchanged and so possibly, the reaction to hyperinsulinism depends on genetic predisposition. There is no doubt that hyperinsulinism influences increased tension of sympathetic systems and on that way may lead to BP increase. Insulin's effect on the vascular wall in HT development should also be mentioned. Under physiological conditions, insulin has a dilating effect on vessels. Nitrogen oxide (NO) mediates in causing this effect, production of which is controlled by enzymatic systems participating in glucose metabolism. As a result of insulin resistance, glucose utilisation is reduced together with NO synthesis, which causes suppression of the vasodilative insulin effect. Insulin also increases endothelin-1 synthesis, which explains why high concentrations indirectly cause a vasoconstrictive effect. Also, insulin intensifies RAAS system activity, intensifies renal sodium reabsorption, has a pro-inflammatory effect, increases release of free fat acids from adipocytes, intensifies oxidation stress and has a mitogenic effect on vessel walls. All these actions lead to BP increase, and also accelerate atherosclerosis development [44].

Adipocytokines and Their Role in HT Combined with Obesity Development

Fat tissue was long considered to be only energy storage, but it also performs endocrine, autocrine and paracrine functions in the body. Expression of many proteins and receptors with key importance for metabolic changes occur in adipocytes (table 1).

One of the best-known proteins produced by adipocytes is **leptin**. Leptin acts via the central nervous system inhibits food intake, regulates secretion of gonadotropin and increases tension in sympathetic systems.

High leptin levels and resistance to leptin has been found in obese people. Experiments on rodents related to exogenous leptin administered intravenously and intraventricularly show an increase in arterial blood pressure [45, 46], which revert after the adrenergic system blockade [47]. Reports on leptin hypertensive effect in people are not so clear.

Rosmond et al. [48] showed that in persons with high BMI and hyperleptinemia, HT appears only when they are carriers of the most common genotype for the leptin receptor. Other, more rarely occurring variations of this receptor seem to protect patients against BP increase.

Table 1. Active substances produced by fat tissue

Substances produced only and almost only in fat tissue	Substances excreted by, amongst others, adipocytes
leptin adiponectin agouti protein visfatin apelin chemerin	TGF-β TNF-α PAI-1 angiotensin renin angiotensin convertase chymase cathepsin D i G prostaglandins (PGI_2, $PGF_{2\alpha}$) resistin IGF-1 VEGEF MIF IL-6 glucocorticoids and sex hormones

This would explain the fact that in the majority of obese persons there is BP increase, but there is a certain group of patients for whom, despite considerable obesity, the pressure value remains normal. Leptin also increases reactive oxygen species (ROS) generation in endothelial cells [49] and stimulates pro-inflammatory cytokine production such as TNF-α, or IL-6 participating in HT and atherosclerosis pathogenesis [50, 51].

A second cytokine produced only by adipocytes is **adiponectin**, which concentration considerably decreases, for example, in obesity. Adiponectin has insulin-sensitizing, anti-inflammatory and anti-atherosclerotic effect. Hypoadiponectinemia causes impaired vessels' relaxation related to endothelium dysfunction, and may result in BP increase [52, 53].

Many authors have shown a relationship between hypoadiponectinemia and higher BP values [54, 55, 56, 57]. An adiponectin stimulating effect on endothelial nitrogen oxide production and on angiogenesis was also proved [58]. Adiponectin's role in inhibiting ICAM-1, VCAM-1 and E-selectin adhesive molecule expression has also been highlighted. Those proteins that are receptors for monocytes induce the atherosclerotic process. Monocytes which adhere to damaged endothelium, penetrate to the subendothelial space, where they capture LDL-cholesterol from circulation and undergo transformation to foam cells [59, 60]. The quoted study suggests that adiponectin inhibits creation of atherosclerotic plaque in the very early stages, and hypoadiponectinemia may be considered a new cardiovascular risk factor.

Resistin's role in CVD pathogenesis in people is not fully explained. After first reports on resistin's role as an adipocytokine in insulin resistance pathogenesis [61, 62, 63], new studies emerged as a result of which final explanations of their effect in people are still far off [64]. It is currently known that a main source of resistin is not fat tissue, as previously believed, but monocytes and macrophage of peripheral blood and the resistin itself participates in inducing inflammatory processes and may be an additional accelerating factor for atherosclerosis development [65].

According to recent studies **visfatin** and **apelin** cytokines produced in fat tissue seem to have a protective function in obese patients. Visfatin regulates Langerhans β cells' functions [66] and reduces the glucose level in blood, while apelin stimulates endothelium-dependent, nitric oxide-mediated vasorelaxation and reduces BP [67], also acting through inhibition of angiotensin II activity [68].

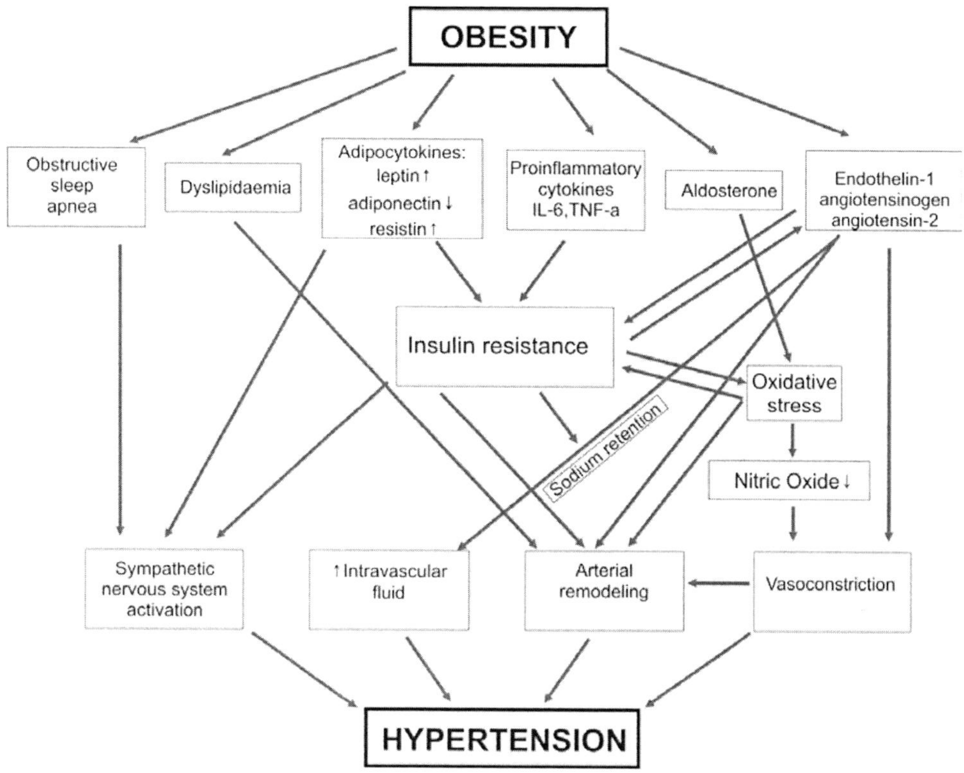

Figure 1. Factors participating in arterial hypertension etiopathogenesis in obese persons.

Pathogenic Relations of Atherosclerosis and Arterial Hypertension

Atherosclerosis clinical symptoms usually reveal themselves after 50 years of age, but it is a progressive process from childhood or the teenage years [69]. In persons of the developmental age, atherosclerosis changes have the character of fatty streaks. These are reversible changes, not causing any complaints. If however, vessel walls shall be exposed to mechanical, chemical or biological effects causing them damage, then fatty infiltration undergoes a gradual transformation into fibrous plaque [70]. Clinical symptoms will depend on location and advancement of the atherosclerosis plaque creation process. Mechanical forces related to blood flow react continuously on the endothelium, and the flow method (laminar, turbulent, and oscillating) influences the type of response in the endothelium [71].

Apart from mechanical factors in endothelium dysfunction, immunological, free radicals and metabolic factors are also responsible, particularly lipoprotein-LDL and VLDL, lipoprotein (a), triglycerides, oxysterols, free fat acids, reactive oxygen/nitrogen species, fibrinogen, C-reactive protein (CRP), cytokines and intracellular adhesion molecule-1 (ICAM-1), and vascular adhesion molecule1 (VCAM-1) [72,73]. A vital role in this process is also played by blood morphotic elements – platelets undergoing excessive adhesion to the damaged endothelium and aggregation [74] and monocytes/ macrophages capturing oxidate modified lipoproteins [75] with the participation of scavenger type receptors and transforming them into foam cells [76]. Among essential risk factors related to atherosclerosis, hyperuricemia [77] and hyperhomocysteinemia [78] are also mentioned.

Atherosclerosis is then a chronic disease with a multifactor etiology. This applies especially to small and medium-sized arteries, and particularly in their branching and bifurcations. In this places because the laminar blood flow undergoes disorder providing appropriate shear stress, stimulating nitric oxide synthesis here. The blood flow method also modifies the gene expression of those participating in atherosclerosis pathogenesis. The afore-mentioned pathomechanisms gain a special meaning in development of atherosclerosis changes in HT persons. Blood pressure on vessel walls and shear stress are increased in those patients, which in a mechanical way damages the endothelium and stimulates the proliferation of smooth vascular muscle cells. Diastolic endothelium activity is then disturbed due to decreased production and increased inactivation of nitrogen oxide. Increased angiotensin II activity stimulates free oxygen radicals, intensifying the inflammation process and endothelium dysfunction [79]. Moreover, it stimulates TGF-β synthesis, excessive production of which effects HT development [80]. In this way the HT makes both an atherosclerosis change initiation factor as well as favouring their progression. Clinical studies confirm the relationship of HT in children and teens with atherosclerosis changes [81], and this is also related to increase of left heart ventricle mass, which is a main hypertension organ complication and at the same time an indicator of the threat of ischemic disease development [82]. A proof for vascular change is the increase of intimae-media complex thickness of common carotid arteries and decreased dilatability of arm arteries after reactive congestion being a result of endothelium function impairment. A positive correlation of BMI with high arterial blood pressure was proved and both obesity and HT are mentioned among atherosclerosis risk factors in children and teenage populations [83, 84, 85]. Activation of the renin-angiotensin-aldosterone system which accompanies obesity effects not only HT development but also has a pro-thrombotic effect on atherosclerosis change progression [86]. It should also be remembered that angiotensiogen synthesis is higher in visceral than subcutaneous fat tissue [87]. Increased homocysteine concentration as a risk factor for atherosclerosis-dependent diseases in adults [88], was also found in obese school children showing HT and dyslipidemia [89]. A higher variable homocysteine concentration was also found in children with a family history of early occurrence of ischemic heart disease [90]. Primary HT more often than secondary is accompanied by hyperuricemia in teens [91]. Uric acid may play the role of antioxidant [92], but in excess it may also have a pro-oxidative effect and epidemiological studies have indicated its relationship with hypertension, metabolic syndromes or coronary heart disease [91].

Excessive food intake increases tension of the sympathetic nervous system [93]. Its activity also increases in relation to insulin resistance and consequent hyperinsulinemia [94], and also under the influence of leptin [95]. Obesity duration time, intensification and fat tissue distribution have a fundamental importance in the cardiological consequences of obesity, in the form of heart dysfunction and hypertrophy of the left ventricle [96]. These are also HT and cardiovascular risk markers [82].

Metabolic Syndrome in Children and Adolescents

Metabolic syndrome (MS) in the adult population defines a syndrome of metabolic and haemodynamic disorders, including visceral obesity, atherogenic dyslipidemia, carbohydrate metabolism disorders such as resistance to insulin and hyperinsulinism, and coexistence of HT. The occurrence of MS features is combined with an increased death risk, sick rate from CVD and type 2 diabetes. With reference to adults there are two MS definitions. The first, published in 1988 in Europe by the World Health Organisation (WHO) defines MS as a coexisting resistance to insulin (expressed by existence of type 2 diabetes or increased fasting glycaemia or glucose intolerance) with at least 2 features from the following: HT during treatment or SBP>140 mmHg and/or DBP> 90 mmHg, dyslipidemia [(triglycerides >150 mg/dl and/or HDL-cholesterol (HDL-ch) <35 mg/dl (men), <40 mg/dl (women)], obesity - BMI≥ 30 kg/m^2 and/or waist to hip ratio (WHR) >0.9 (men) and >0.85 (women), or albumin with urine discharge > 20 μg/min or >30 mg/1 g of creatinine [97]. A second definition established in the USA by the Third Adult Treatment Panel of the National Cholesterol Education Program (NCEP-ATP III) requires coexistence of at least 3 out of five of these anomalies: abdominal obesity (waist circumference ≥ 94 cm in men and ≥ 80 cm in women), triglyceride level ≥ 150 mg/dl, HDL-ch ≤ 40 mg/dl in men, ≤ 50 mg/dl in women, fasting glycaemia ≥ 110 mg/dl [98]. In 2005 the International Diabetes Federation prepared new, practical MS diagnosis criteria based on which diagnosis of MS requires the following findings: abdominal obesity (border waist circumference changes according to ethnic group) and additionally, at least two out of four of these features: triglyceride level ≥ 150 mg/dl, HDL-ch ≤ 40 mg/dl in men and ≤ 50 mg/dl in women or dyslipidemia treatment; BP ≥ 130/85 or HT treatment and fasting glycemia ≥ 100 mg/dl or type 2 diabetes treatment. We still require an MS definition for the child and teenage populations. Individual authors in their reports use various reference criteria and standards in defining MS in patients from this age group (table 2).

The MS occurrence frequency in the child/teen population is difficult to evaluate due to the considerable difference in cut-off points (standards) selection used by the researchers. For Goodman et al. [106], the MS occurrence frequency in school children evaluates to 4.2% to 8.4% depending on the MS definition used (NCEP vs. WHO). The Bogalusa Heart Study [107] analysis showed that MS features occur with a 3.6% frequency in a teen group of 8 - 17 years of age. In our own studies in Polish children, MS features were found in 25% of patients with primary HT [108] and in 55% with simple obesity [109]. Similar results were also obtained by Weiss et al. [103] who found MS features in 50% of obese children, and Litwin [110] who found MS in 20% of children and teens with primary HT. Upon analysis of the results of numerous studies, it may be stated that MS is a multi-system risk factor for cardiovascular disease [111]. However, unclear and incomplete criteria still create much controversy without considering many factors having a significant effect on CVD risk evaluation (e.g. age, smoking, life style, family history), without the heaviness, advancement and importance of each criteria's assessment. But there is no doubt that coexistence of obesity and HT (integral MS components) in children and teenager increases the risk of early atherosclerosis development and the occurrence of atherosclerosis-dependent diseases. Therefore it is vital to include those young persons in appropriate procedures [112]. Due to the disturbing growth in the frequency of occurrence in children and teens of both obesity and obesity coexisting with HT, it is a vital task for public health educators [113].

Table 2. Definitions for metabolic syndrome in children (cut-off points)

Author, year	Glucose tolerance	Obesity	Triglycerides	HDL-ch	BP
Srinivasan et al. 2002 [99]	fasting insulin $\geq$ P -75th	BMI $\geq$ P-75th	ratios TCh/HDL-ch or TAG/HDL-ch $\geq$ P-75th		$\geq$ P-75th
Cook et al. 2003 [100]	fasting glucose $\geq$ 100 mg/dl	WC > P-90th	$\geq$ 110 mg/dl	$\leq$ 40 mg/dl	$\geq$ P-90th
de Ferranti et al. 2004 [101]	fasting glucose $\geq$ 110 mg/dl	WC > P-75th	$\geq$ 100 mg/dl	$\leq$ 50 mg/dl	> P-90th
Cruz et al. 2004 [102]	fasting glucose $\geq$ 110 and <126 mg/dl	WC $\geq$ P-90th	$\geq$ P-90th	$\leq$ P-10th	> P-90th
Weiss et al. 2004 [103]	glucose $\geq$ 140 mg/dl at 2h	BMI – Z score $\geq$ 2,0	> P-95th	< P-5th	> P-95th
Lambert et al. 2004 [104]	5,9-6,1 mmol/l	WC $\geq$ P-95th	M $\geq$ 0,9 mmol/l F $\geq$ 1,0 mmol/l	$\leq$ P- 5th	$\geq$ P-95th
Ford et al. 2005 [105]	fasting glucose $\geq$ 110 mg/dl	WC $\geq$ P-90th	$\geq$ 110 mg/dl	$\leq$ 40 mg/dl	$\geq$ P-90th

Abbreviations: P – percentiles for age and gender, BMI – body mass index, WC – waist circumference, TCh – total cholesterol, HDL-ch – HDL-cholesterol, TAG – triglycerides, M – male, F – female, BP – blood pressure.

References

[1] Barlow SE, Dietz WH. Obesity evaluation and treatment: Expert Committee recommendations. The Maternal and Child Health Bureau, Health Resources and Services Administration and the Department of Health and Human Services. *Pediatrics*. 1998;102(3): E29.

[2] Zhang C, Rexrode KM, van Dam RM, Li TY, Hu FB. Abdominal obesity and the risk of all-cause, cardiovascular, and cancer mortality: sixteen years of follow-up in US women. *Circulation.* 2008; 117(13): 1658-67.

[3] Maziak W, Ward KD, Stockton MB Childhood obesity: are we missing the big picture? *Obes Rev.* 2008, 9: 35–42.

[4] Calle EE, Thun MJ, Petrelli JM, Rodriguez C, Heath CW Jr. Body-mass index and mortality in a prospective cohort of U.S. adults. *N. Engl. J. Med.* 1999; 341(15): 1097-105.

[5] World Health Organization, Global strategy on diet, physical activity and health. http://www.who.int/dietphysicalactivity/publications/facts/obesity/en/.

[6] Currie C, Roberts C, Morgan A, Smith R, Settertobulte W, Samdal O, Barnekow V, Rasmussen., eds. Young people's health in context. Health Behaviour in School-aged Children (HBSC) study: international report from the 2001/2002 survey. Copenhagen, WHO Regional Office for Europe, 2004 (Health Policy for Children and Adolescents, No. 4; http://www.euro.who.int/Document/e82923.

[7] Canoy D, Buchan I. Challenges in obesity epidemiology. *Obes. Rev.* 2007, Suppl 1:1-11.

[8] Al-Haddad FH, Little BB, Abdul Ghafoor AG. Childhood obesity in United Arab Emirates schoolchildren: a national study. *Ann. Hum. Biol.* 2005; 32(1): 72-9.

[9] Nelson JA, Chiasson MA, Ford V. Childhood overweight in a New York City WIC population. *Am. J. Public Health* 2004; 94: 458-62.

[10] Freedman DS, Khan LK, Serdula MK, Dietz WH, Srinivasan SR, Berenson GS. The relation of childhood BMI to adult adiposity: the Bogalusa Heart Study. *Pediatrics.* 2005; 115: 22-7.

[11] Małecka-Tendera E, Klimek K, Matusik P, Olszanecka-Glinianowicz M., Lehingue Y, on behalf of the Polish Childhood Obesity Study Group. Obesity and overweight prevalence in Polish 7-to 9-year-old children. *Obes. Res.* 2005; 13: 964–968.

[12] Kelly T, Yang W, Chen CS, Reynolds K, He J. Global burden of obesity in 2005 and projections to 2030. *Int J Obes* (Lond). 2008, www.nature.com/ijo.

[13] Poirier P, Giles TD, Bray GA, Hong Y, Stern JS, Pi-Sunyer FX, Eckel RH; American Heart Association; Obesity Committee of the Council on Nutrition, Physical Activity, and Metabolism. Obesity and cardiovascular disease: pathophysiology, evaluation, and effect of weight loss: an update of the 1997 American Heart Association Scientific Statement on Obesity and Heart Disease from the Obesity Committee of the Council on Nutrition, Physical Activity, and Metabolism. *Circulation.* 2006, 14; 113(6): 898-918.

[14] Chobanian AV, Bakris GL, Black HR, Cushman WC, Green LA, Izzo JL Jr, Jones DW, Materson BJ, Oparil S, Wright JT Jr, Roccella EJ; National Heart, Lung, and Blood Institute Joint National Committee on Prevention, Detection, Evaluation, and Treatment of High Blood Pressure; National High Blood Pressure Education Program Coordinating Committee. The Seventh Report of the Joint National Committee on Prevention, Detection, Evaluation, and Treatment of High Blood Pressure: the JNC 7 report. *JAMA.* 2003; 289: 2560–2572.

[15] World Health Report 2002: Reducing risks, promoting healthy life. Geneva, Switzerland: World Health Organization, 2002. http://www.who.int/whr/2002.

[16] Sorof JM, Lai D, Turner J, Poffenbarger T, Portman RJ. Overweight, ethnicity, and the prevalence of hypertension in school-aged children. *Pediatrics*. 2004; 113(3 Pt 1): 475-482.

[17] Bryl W, Miczke A, Pupek-Musialik D. Hypertension and obesity – increasing problem of young patients. *Endokrynologia, Otyłość i Zaburzenia Przemiany Materii*, 2005; 1 (1):: 26-29.

[18] Moore WE, Stephens A, Wilson T, Wilson W, Eichner JE. Body mass index and blood pressure screening in a rural public school system: the Healthy Kids Project. *Prev Chronic Dis*. 2006; 3(4): A114.

[19] Rosner B, Prineas R, Daniels SR, Loggie J. Blood pressure differences between blacks and whites in relation to body size among US children and adolescents. *Am. J. Epidemiol*. 2000, 15; 151(10): 1007-19.

[20] Freedman DS, Dietz WH, Srinivasan SR, Berenson GS. The relation of overweight to cardiovascular risk factors among children and adolescents: the Bogalusa Heart Study. *Pediatrics*. 1999; 103 (6 Pt 1): 1175-82.

[21] Sorof JM, Poffenbarger T, Franco K, Bernard L, Portman RJ. Isolated systolic hypertension, obesity, and hyperkinetic hemodynamic states in children. *J. Pediatr*. 2002; 140(6): 643-5.

[22] Fogelholm M, van Marken Lichtenbelt W. Comparison of body composition methods: a literature analysis. *Eur. J. Clin. Nutr*. 1997; 51: 495–503.

[23] National Institutes of Health, National Heart, Lung and Blood Institute. Obesity education initiative: clinical guidelines on the identification, evaluation, and treatment of overweight and obesity in adults. The Evidence Report: US Department of Health and Human Services, Public Health Service, NIH, HHLBI. Bethesda, Md 1998.

[24] National High Blood Pressure Education Program Working Group on High Blood Pressure in Children and Adolescents. The fourth report on the diagnosis, evaluation, and treatment of high blood pressure in children and adolescents. *Pediatrics* 2004; 114: 555–76.

[25] Metoki H, Ohkubo T, Kikuya M, Asayama K, Obara T, Hara A, Hirose T, Hashimoto J, Totsune K, Hoshi H, Satoh H, Imai Y. Prognostic significance of night-time, early morning, and daytime blood pressures on the risk of cerebrovascular and cardiovascular mortality: the Ohasama Study. *J. Hypertens*. 2006; 24: 1841–1848.

[26] Graves JW, Althaf MM. Utility of ambulatory blood pressure monitoring in children and adolescents. *Pediatr Nephrol*. 2006; 21: 1640 –1652.

[27] Urbina E, Alpert B, Flynn J, Hayman L, Harshfield GA, Jacobson M, Mahoney L, McCrindle B, Mietus-Snyder M, Steinberger J, Daniels S; American Heart Association Atherosclerosis, Hypertension, and Obesity in Youth Committee. Ambulatory blood pressure monitoring in children and adolescents: recommendations for standard assessment: a scientific statement from the American Heart Association Atherosclerosis, Hypertension, and Obesity in Youth Committee of the council on cardiovascular disease in the young and the council for high blood pressure research. *Hypertension*. 2008; 52(3): 433-451.

[28] Garrison RJ, Kannel WB, Stokes J 3rd, Castelli WP. Incidence and precursors of hypertension in young adults: the Framingham Offspring Study. *Prev. Med.* 1987; 16(2): 235-51.

[29] Pihlajamäki J, Gylling H, Miettinen TA, Laakso M. Insulin resistance is associated with increased cholesterol synthesis and decreased cholesterol absorption in normoglycemic men. *J. Lipid. Res.* 2004; 45: 507–512.

[30] Adeli K, Taghibiglou C, Van Iderstine SC, Lewis GF. Mechanisms of hepatic very low-density lipoprotein overproduction in insulin resistance. *Trends Cardiovasc Med.* 2001, 11: 170–176.

[31] Tobin KA, Ulven SM, Schuster GU, Steineger HH, Andresen SM, Gustafsson JA, Nebb HI. Liver x receptors as insulin-mediating factors in fatty acid and cholesterol biosynthesis. *J. Biol. Chem.* 2002; 277: 10691–10697.

[32] Nishina M, Kikuchi T, Yamazaki H, Kameda K, Hiura M, Uchiyama M. Relationship among systolic blood pressure, serum insulin and leptin, and visceral fat accumulation in obese children. *Hypertens Res.* 2003; 26(4):281-8.

[33] Maffeis C, Pietrobelli A, Grezzani A, Provera S, Tatò L. Waist circumference and cardiovascular risk factors in prepubertal children. *Obes. Res.* 2001; 9(3):179-87.

[34] Fox CS, Massaro JM, Hoffmann U, Pou KM, Maurovich-Horvat P, Liu CY, Vasan RS, Murabito JM, Meigs JB, Cupples LA, D'Agostino RB Sr, O'Donnell CJ. Abdominal visceral and subcutaneous adipose tissue compartments: association with metabolic risk factors in the Framingham Heart Study. *Circulation.* 2007, 3; 116(1):39-48.

[35] Julius S, Valentini M, Palatini P. Overweight and hypertension: a 2-way street? *Hypertension* 2000; 35: 807–813.

[36] Davy KP, Hall JE.. Obesity and hypertension: two epidemics or one? *Am. J. Physiol. Regul. Integr. Comp. Physiol.* 2004; 286: R803–R813.

[37] Jiang X, Srinivasan SR, Urbina E, Berenson GS. Hyperdynamic circulation and cardiovascular risk in children and adolescents: the Bogalusa Heart Study. *Circulatio.* 1995; 91:1101–1106.

[38] Hall JE, Brands MW, Dixon WN, Smith MJ Jr. Obesity-induced hypertension. Renal function and systemic hemodynamics. *Hypertension* 1993; 22(3):292-9.

[39] Esler M. On a low calorie diet, are there separate and discrete effects of negative energy balance and weight loss on blood pressure? *J. Hypertens* 2003; 21: 261–262.

[40] Goodfriend TL, Kelley DE, Goodpaster BH, Winters SJ. Visceral obesity and insulin resistance are associated with plasma aldosterone levels in women. *Obes. Res.* 1999; 7(4): 355-62.

[41] Bloomfield GL, Sugerman HJ, Blocher CR, Gehr TW, Sica DA. Chronically increased intra-abdominal pressure produces systemic hypertension in dogs. *Int. J. Obes. Relat. Metab. Disord.* 2000; 24(7): 819-24.

[42] Hall JE. Mechanisms of abnormal renal sodium handling in obesity hypertension. Am. *J. Hypertens.* 1997; 10(5 Pt 2): 49S-55S.

[43] DuRant RH, Baranowski T, Rhodes T, Gutin B, Thompson WO, Carroll R, Puhl J, Greaves KA. Association among serum lipid and lipoprotein concentrations and physical activity, physical fitness, and body composition in young children. *J. Pediatr.* 1993; 123(2):185-92.

[44] Muniyappa R, Montagnani M, Koh KK, Quon MJ. Cardiovascular actions of insulin. *Endocr Rev*. 2007; 28(5): 463-91

[45] Shek EW, Brands MW, Hall JE. Chronic leptin infusion increases arterial pressure. *Hypertension* 1998; 31: 409–414.

[46] Correia ML, Morgan DA, Sivitz WI, Mark AL, Haynes WG. Leptin acts in the central nervous system to produce dose– dependent changes in arterial pressure. *Hypertension* 2001;37: 936 –942.

[47] Carlyle M, Jones OB, Kuo JJ, Hall JE. Chronic cardiovascular and renal actions of leptin: role of adrenergic activity. *Hypertension* 2002; 39: 496–501.

[48] Rosmond R, Chagnon YC, Holm G, Chagnon M, Pérusse L, Lindell K, Carlsson B, Bouchard C, Björntorp P.. Hypertension in obesity and the leptin receptor gene locus. *J. Clin. Endocrinol. Metab*. 2000; 85: 3126–3131.

[49] Bouloumie A, Marumo T, Lafontan M, Busse R. Leptin induces oxidative stress in human endothelial cells. *FASEB J*. 1999; 13: 1231–1238.

[50] Navarro J, Redon J, Cea-Calvo L, Lozano JV, Fernandez-Perez C, Bonet A, Gonzalez-Esteban J. Metabolic syndrome, organ damage and cardiovascular disease in treated hypertensive patients. the ERIC-HTA study. *Blood Press*. 2007; 16: 20 –27.

[51] Cuspidi C, Meani S, Fusi V, Severgnini B, Valerio C, Catini E, Leonetti G, Magrini F, Zanchetti A. Metabolic syndrome and target organ damage in untreated essential hypertensives. *J. Hypertens*. 2004; 22: 1991–1998.

[52] Tan KC, Xu A, Chow WS, Lam MC, Ai VH, Tam SC, Lam KS. Hypoadiponectinaemia is associated with impaired endothelium-dependant vasodilatation. *J. Clin. Endocrinol. Metab*. 2004; 89(2): 765–769.

[53] Shimabukuro M, Higa N, Asahi T, Oshiro Y, Takasu N, Tagawa T, Ueda S, Shimomura I, Funahashi T, Matsuzawa Y. Hypoadiponectinaemia is closely linked to endothelial dysfunction in man. *J. Clin. Endocrinol. Metab*. 2003; 88(7): 3236–3240.

[54] Hong SJ, Park CG, Seo HS, Oh DJ, Ro YM. Associations among plasma adiponectin, hypertension, left ventricular diastolic function and left ventricular mass index. *Blood Press* 2004; 13(4): 236–242.

[55] Lee HS, Lee M, Joung H. Adiponectin represents an independent risk factor for hypertension in middle aged Korean women. *Asia Pac. J. Clin. Nutr*. 2007; 16(1): 10–15.

[56] Chow WS, Cheung BM, Tso AW, Xu A, Wat NM, Fong CH, Ong LH, Tam S, Tan KC, Janus ED, Lam TH, Lam KS. Hypoadiponectinemia as a predictor for the development of hypertension: a 5-year prospective study. *Hypertension* 2007; 49(6): 1455–1461.

[57] Murakami H, Ura N, Furuhashi M, Higashiura K, Miura T, Shimamoto K. Role of adiponectin in insulin-resistant hypertension and atherosclerosis. *Hypertens Res*. 2003; 26(9): 705–710.

[58] Chen H, Montagnani M, Funahashi T, Shimomura I, Quon MJ.. Adiponectin stimulates production of nitric oxide in vascular endothelial cells. *J. Biol. Chem*. 2003; 278(45): 45021–45026.

[59] Ouchi N, Kihara S, Arita Y, Maeda K, Kuriyama H, Okamoto Y, Hotta K, Nishida M, Takahashi M, Nakamura T, Yamashita S, Funahashi T, Matsuzawa Y. Novel modulator

for endothelial adhesion molecules: adipocyte-derived plasma protein adiponectin. *Circulation* 1999; 100(25): 2473–2476.

[60] Ouchi N, Kihara S, Arita Y, Nishida M, Matsuyama A, Okamoto Y, Ishigami M, Kuriyama H, Kishida K, Nishizawa H, Hotta K, Muraguchi M, Ohmoto Y, Yamashita S, Funahashi T, Matsuzawa Y. Adipocyte-derived plasma protein, adiponectin, suppresses lipid accumulation and class A scavenger receptor expression in human monocyte-derived macrophages. *Circulation* 2001; 103(8); 1057–1063.

[61] Azuma K, Katsukawa F, Oguchi S, Murata M, Yamazaki H, Shimada A, Saruta T. Correlation between serum resistin level and adiposity in obese individuals. *Obes. Res.* 2003; 11(8): 997-1001.

[62] Zhang JL, Qin YW, Zheng X, Qie JL, Zou DJ. Serum resistin level in essential hypertension patients with different glucose tolerance. *Diabet Med.* 2003; 20:828 –31.

[63] Fujinami A, Obayashi H, Ohta K, Ichimura T, Nishimura M, Matsui H, Kawahara Y, Yamazaki M, Ogata M, Hasegawa G, Nakamura N, Yoshikawa T, Nakano K, Ohta M. Enzyme-linked immunosorbent assay for circulating human resistin: resistin concentrations in normal subjects and patients with type 2 diabetes. *Clin. Chim. Acta.* 2004; 339(1-2): 57-63.

[64] Silha JV, Krsek M, Skrha JV, Sucharda P, Nyomba BLG, Murphy LJ. Plasma resistin, adiponection and leptin levels in lean and obese subjects: correlations with insulin resistance. *Eur. J. Endocrinol.* 2003; 149: 331–5.

[65] Reilly MP, Lehrke M, Wolfe ML, Rohatgi A, Lazar MA, Rader DJ. Resistin is an inflammatory marker of atherosclerosis in humans. *Circulation* 2005; 111(7): 932-9.

[66] Rabe K, Lehrke M, Parhofer KG, Broedl UC. Adipokines and insulin resistance. *Mol. Med.* 2008; 14(11-12): 741-51.

[67] Tatemoto K, Takayama K, Zou MX, Kumaki I, Zhang W, Kumano K, Fujimiya M. The novel peptide apelin lowers blood pressure via a nitric oxide-dependent mechanism. *Regul. Pept.* 2001; 99(2-3): 87-92.

[68] Chun HJ, Ali ZA, Kojima Y, Kundu RK, Sheikh AY, Agrawal R, Zheng L, Leeper NJ, Pearl NE, Patterson AJ, Anderson JP, Tsao PS, Lenardo MJ, Ashley EA, Quertermous T. Apelin signaling antagonizes Ang II effects in mouse models of atherosclerosis. *J. Clin. Invest.* 2008;118(10): 3343-54.

[69] Daniels SR, Greer FR, and the Committee on Nutrition. Lipid Screening and cardiovascular health in childhood. *Pediatrics* 2008; 122: 198-208.

[70] Berenson GS, Srinivasan SR, Bao W, Newman WP 3rd, Tracy RE, Wattigney WA. Association between multiple cardiovascular risk factors and the early development of atherosclerosis. Bogalusa Heart Study. *N. Engl. J. Med.* 1998; 338(23): 1650-6.

[71] Brooks AR, Lelkes PI, Rubanyi GM. Gene expression profiling of vascular endothelium cells exposed to fluid mechanical forces: relevance for focal susceptibility to atherosclerosis. *Endothelium* 2004; 11(1): 45-57.

[72] dos Santos MG, Pegoraro M, Sandrini F, Macuco EC. Risk factors for the development of atherosclerosis in childhood and adolescence. *Arq. Bras. Cardiol.* 2008; 90(4): 276-283.

[73] Beauloye V, Zech F, Tran HT, Clapuyt P, Maes M, Brichard SM. Determinants of early atherosclerosis in obese children and adolescents. *J. Clin. Endocrinol. Metab.* 2007; 92(8): 3025-32.

[74] Sorof J, Daniels S. Obesity hypertension in children, a problem of epidemic proportions. *Hypertension* 2002; 40, 441-447.

[75] Libby P, Aikawa M, Schönbeck U. Cholesterol and atherosclerosis. *Biochim. Biophys. Acta.* 2000; 1529(1-3): 299-309.

[76] Falk E. Pathogenesis of atherosclerosis. J Am Coll Cardiol. 2006; 47(8 Suppl): C7-12.

[77] Feig DI, Kang DH, Johnson RJ. Uric acid and cardiovascular risk. *N. Engl. J. Med.* 2008; 359(17): 1811-21.

[78] Scott CH, Sutton MS. Homocysteine: evidence for a causal relationship with cardiovascular disease. *Cardiol. Rev.* 1999; 7(2): 101-7.

[79] Sowers JR. Hypertension, angiotensin II and oxidative stress. *N. Engl. J. Med.* 2002; 346(25): 1999-2001.

[80] August P, Suthanthiran M. Transforming growth factor β signaling, vascular remodeling, and hypertension. *N. Engl. J. Med.* 2006; 354(25): 2721-3.

[81] Hennekens CH. Screening individuals and families with premature coronary heart disease: a clinical and public health challenge. *Eur. Heart J.* 2003; 24(3): 212-3.

[82] Sorof JM, Turner J, Martin DS, Garcia K, Garami Z, Alexandrov AV, Wan F, Portman RJ. Cardiovascular risk factors and sequelae in hypertensive children identified by referral versus school-based screening. *Hypertension.* 2004; 43(2): 214-8.

[83] He Q, Ding ZY, Fong DY, Karlberg J. Blood pressure is associated with body mass index in both normal and obese children. *Hypertension.* 2000; 36(2): 165-70.

[84] Paradis G, Lambert M, O'Loughlin J, Lavallée C, Aubin J, Delvin E, Lévy E. Hanley JA. Blood pressure and adiposity in children and adolescents. *Circulation.* 2004; 110(13): 1832-8.

[85] dos Santos MG, Pegoraro M, Sandrini F, Macuco EC. Risk factors for the development of atherosclerosis in childhood and adolescence. *Arq. Bras. Cardiol.* 2008; 90(4): 276-283.

[86] Lip GY. Hypertension and the prothrombotic state *J. Hum. Hypertens.* 2000; 14 (10-11): 687-90.

[87] van Harmelen V, Elizalde M, Ariapart P, Bergstedt-Lindqvist S, Reynisdottir S, Hoffstedt J, Lundkvist I, Bringman S, Arner P. The association of human adipose angiotensinogen gene expression with abdominal fat distribution in obesity. *Int. J. Obes. Relat. Metab. Disord.* 2000; 24(6): 673-8.

[88] Wald DS, Law M, Morris JK. Homocysteine and cardiovascular disease: evidence on causality from a meta-analysis. *BMJ.* 2002; 325(7374): 1202.

[89] Zhu W, Huang X, Li M, Neubauer H. Elevated plasma homocysteine in obese schoolchildren with early atherosclerosis. *Eur. J. Pediatr.* 2006; 165(5): 326-31.

[90] Groner JA, Joshi M, Bauer JA. Pediatric precursors of adult cardiovascular disease: noninvasive assessment of early vascular changes in children and adolescents. *Pediatrics* 2006; 118(4): 1683-91.

[91] Feig DI, Johnson RJ. Hyperuricemia in childhood primary hypertension. *Hypertension* 2003; 42(3): 247-52.

[92] Waring WS, McKnight JA, Webb DJ, Maxwell SR. Uric acid restores endothelial function in patients with type 1 diabetes and regular smokers. *Diabetes* 2006; 55(11): 3127-32.

[93] Hausberg M, Hoffman RP, Somers VK, Sinkey CA, Mark AL, Anderson EA. Contrasting autonomic and hemodynamic effects of insulin in healthy elderly versus young subjects. *Hypertension* 1997; 29(3): 700-5.

[94] Landsberg L. Insulin-mediated sympathetic stimulation: role in the pathogenesis of obesity-related hypertension (or, how insulin affects blood pressure, and why). *J. Hypertens.* 2001; 19(3 Pt 2): 523-8.

[95] Hall JE, Hildebrandt DA, Kuo J. Obesity hypertension: role of leptin and sympathetic nervous system. *Am. J. Hypertens.* 2001; 14(6 Pt 2): 103S-115S.

[96] Gates PE, Gentile CL, Seals DR, Christou DD. Adiposity contributes to differences in left ventricular structure and diastolic function with age in healthy men. *J. Clin. Endocrinol. Metab.* 2003; 88(10): 4884-90.

[97] Alberti KG, Zimmet PZ. Definition, diagnosis and classification of diabetes mellitus and its complications. Part 1: diagnosis and classification of diabetes mellitus provisional report of a WHO consultation. *Diabet Med.* 1998; 15(7): 539-53.

[98] Third Report of the National Cholesterol Education Program (NCEP) Expert Panel on detection, evaluation and treatment of high cholesterol in adults (Adult Treatment Panel III). Final Report. http://www.nhlbi.nih.gov/guidelines/cholesterol/atp3full.pdf.

[99] Srinivasan SR, Myers L, Berenson GS. Predictability of childhood adiposity and insulin for developing insulin resistance syndrome (syndrome X) in young adulthood: the Bogalusa Heart Study. *Diabetes* 2002; 51(1): 204-9.

[100] Cook S, Weitzman M, Auinger P, Nguyen M, Dietz WH. Prevalence of a metabolic syndrome phenotype in adolescents: findings from the third National Health and Nutrition Examination Survey, 1988-1994. *Arch. Pediatr. Adolesc. Med.* 2003; 157(8): 821-7.

[101] de Ferranti SD, Gauvreau K, Ludwig DS, Neufeld EJ, Newburger JW, Rifai N. Prevalence of the metabolic syndrome in American adolescents: findings from the Third National Health and Nutrition Examination Survey. *Circulation* 2004; 110(16): 2494-7.

[102] Cruz ML, Weigensberg MJ, Huang TT, Ball G, Shaibi GQ, Goran MI. The metabolic syndrome in overweight Hispanic youth and the role of insulin sensitivity. *J. Clin. Endocrinol Metab.* 2004; 89(1): 108-13.

[103] Weiss R, Dziura J, Burgert TS, Tamborlane WV, Taksali SE, Yeckel CW, Allen K, Lopes M, Savoye M, Morrison J, Sherwin RS, Caprio S. Obesity and the metabolic syndrome in children and adolescents. *N. Engl. J. Med* 2004; 350: 2362–74.

[104] Lambert M, Paradis G, O'Loughlin J, Delvin EE, Hanley JA, Levy E. Insulin resistance syndrome in a representative sample of children and adolescents from Quebec, Canada. *Int. J. Obes. Relat. Metab. Disord.* 2004; 28(7): 833-41.

[105] Ford ES, Ajani UA, Mokdad AH; National Health and Nutrition Examination. The metabolic syndrome and concentrations of C-reactive protein among U.S. youth. *Diabetes Care* 2005; 28(4): 878-81.

[106] Goodman E, Daniels SR, Meigs JB, Dolan LM. Instability in the diagnosis of metabolic syndrome in adolescents. *Circulation* 2007; 115: 2316-2322.

[107] Srinivasan SR, Myers L, Berenson GS. Predictability of childhood adiposity and insulin for developing insulin resistance syndrome (syndrome X) in young adulthood: the Bogalusa Heart Study. *Diabetes* 2002; 51(1): 204-9.

[108] Kniażewska MH, Żmudzińska-Kitczak J, Urban K, Obuchowicz AK, Niwińska-Faryna B, Pietrzak JA, Świętochowska-Chechlińska AA, Głowacki JG. Characteristics of metabolic syndrome in children and adolescents with arterial hypertension. *Wiad Lek.* 2005; 58 Suppl 1: 25-8.

[109] Kniażewska MH, Obuchowicz AK, Żmudzińska-Kitczak J, Urban K, Marek M, Zeckei J, Wierzyk A. Cechy zespołu metabolicznego u dzieci i młodzieży z otyłością prostą. *Endokrynologia, Otyłość i Zaburzenia Przemiany Materii* 2007; 3(2): 96.

[110] Litwin M, Sladowska J, Antoniewicz J, Niemirska A, Wierzbicka A, Daszkowska J, Wawer ZT, Janas R, Grenda R. Metabolic abnormalities, insulin resistance, and metabolic syndrome in children with primary hypertension. *Am. J. Hypertens.* 2007; 20(8): 875-82.

[111] Kahn R, Buse J, Ferrannini E, Stern M; American Diabetes Association; European Association for the Study of Diabetes. The metabolic syndrome: time for a critical appraisal: joint statement from the American Diabetes Association and the European Association for the Study of Diabetes. *Diabetes Care.* 2005; 28(9): 2289-304.

[112] American Heart Association Guidlines for primary prevention of atherosclerosis cardiovascular disease begining in childhood. *Circulation* 2003; 107: 1562-1566.

[113] McMahan CA, Gidding SS, Malcom GT, Tracy RE, Strong JP, McGill HC Jr; Pathobiological Determinants of Atherosclerosis in Youth Research Group. Pathobiological determinants of atherosclerosis in youth risk scores are associated with early and advanced atherosclerosis. *Pediatrics* 2006; 118(4): 1447-55.

In: Hypertension, Heredity and Stroke
Editor: Cristina Moratinos and Bruno Cardenas
ISBN 978-1-60741-496-4

Chapter 3

On the Existing Relationships between the Physical Activity, Tobacco Consumption, Body Composition and Socioeconomic Status as a Function of the Blood Pressure smong Spanish Adolescents

***Cordente Martínez, A. Carlos* [1], *García Soidán Pilar*[2], *Sillero Quintana, Manuel*[1], *Stirling James*[1]**
[1]Faculty of sciences of the physical activity and sports.
Polytechnic University of Madrid
[2]Faculty of social sciences and communication.
University of Vigo (Spain)

Abstract

After obtaining a written consent of the parents, subjects from ages 13 to 17 were studied in a representative sample of 474 subjects, 204 boys and 270 girls from 35 educative centres (18 privates and 17 publics) from 16 of the 21 districts of the city of Madrid.

It was found that 12.7% of the boys and 35.6% of the girls were inactive or sedentary. The socioeconomic status significantly determined the physical activity of the girls, especially in the age group 16-17. The girls had a tobacco consumption significantly superior to the boys. A significant inverse relation of the tobacco consumption with the physical activity was found for boys. 47.4% of the girls of the sample were lightly overweight to obese as opposed to the 14.7% of boys. A significant association between adiposity and physical activity in the girls was observed.

The averages for the systolic/diastolic blood pressure were 125.6/71.3 mmHg in boys and 118/69.4 mmHg in girls. A significant relation between the gender and the systolic blood pressure was found.

Solely one relation was found between the blood pressure and the others studied variables: the relation between the physical activity and the diastolic blood pressure for boys (69.9 mmHg for active or very active and 74.1 mmHg for moderately active to sedentary).

As a result of our observations the following series of proposals for the future were made:

The lack of existing relations between the blood pressure and the others variables support the hypothesis that the the effects of these variables on the cardiovascular risk factors needs a longer term to be obvious. Then, it seems to be necessary to suggest future longitudinal studies to know exactly the influence of the healthy habits on the blood pressure of children and adolescents.

Furthermore, girls and subjects from the lower socioeconomico status should receive high-priority attention concerning the health-related habits as physical activity, tobacco consumption or dietary habits which could have a great influence in the future on the blood pressure and other cardiovascular risk factors.

Introduction

Cardiovascular diseases, including arterial hypertension, are the main cause of mortality, morbidity, disability, low productivity and medical costs in industrialized societies [35,36,60,61]. Spain does not escape this pattern: in 1999, 35.5% of the deaths (the primary cause of mortality in Spain) were due to diseases of the circulatory apparatus [30]. In relation to morbidity the same institution indicates that, in 1999, 13.7% of hospital stays had to do with cardiovascular diseases.

In a study in the urban area of Madrid, it was found that 41% of chronic patients in a disability situation were diagnosed with cardiovascular diseases. More than half of them corresponded to a cerebrovascular accident, the disease most closely associated with the arterial hypertension [8].

Currently, hypertension represents a problem and a challenge for public health in Spain due to its high prevalence: around 35% of the adult population, 43% between 35 and 65 years and 56% in people of 60 years or more [9]. This disease also has a series of social repercussions that can effect both the individuals' professional and family environment.

Hypertension has great economic repercussions as far as the welfare cost of the patient (ambulatory and hospital), pharmaceutical cost and related costs due to premature deaths (25% of the total of deaths and 40% of the due ones to cardiovascular diseases in Spain) and related incapacities. Between 1995 and 2001 in Spain, the cost in antihypertensive drugs increased by 61.7% hence as a result in 2001 antihypertensive drugs accounted for 14.3% of the total national health systems pharmaceutical cost. These data do not include, intra-hospitable consumption, private consumption or consumption in non public insuring organizations, nor the consumption of medicine without prescription or that excluded from financing by the national health system [23]. It is estimated that in Spain, the number of patients under antihypertensive treatment surpasses 6% of the population [24]. As a result it is obvious that it is one of the pathologies of greater clinical importance with both social and economic repercussion.

A great number of epidemiological studies [15,53,61] have agreed that the individuals with the greatest risk of suffering arteriosclerosis due to non genetic reasons are those in which we observed one or several of the following risk factors:

- Hypercholesterolemia
- Hypertension
- Tobacco consumption.

These risk factors are associated with the following conditions:

- Obesity.
- Diabetes.
- Bad dietary practice.
- Sedentary and/or stressed lifestyle.

Therefore, some of the major risk factors for the coronary disease are related to the lifestyle. As a result such factors are potentially modifiable [21,50,60]. These modifiable factors include diet, tobacco consumption and physical activity. When an individual has more than one of these risk factors, the probabilities of suffering a vascular accident could be multiplied by up to 16 times [53].

The exact aetiology of hypertension is not known but it is attributed to genetic and/or environmental factors [15,21]. The environmental factors related to hypertension include excessive sodium ingestion, excessive weight, tobacco consumption and physical inactivity. As a result of this, the strategies for intervention and prevention in children have focused, apart from the pharmacological therapy, on their diet, tobacco consumption and physical exercise (essentially aerobic) [15,16,21].

With respect to body composition, the relative amount of fat is the measurement most common in adults and children due to the well established relation between body fat, fitness, athletic performance and endocrine and nutritional alterations [33].

Obesity and overweight are of great interest for public health, because of their association with the increased risk of coronary diseases, hypertension, diabetes and some cancers, etc. [15,26]. The frequency of obesity is increasing alarmingly in the developed countries [15,37,39,43] reaching 39% in the U.S.A. in the last 20 years [49]. Obesity in adolescents is significantly related to that in adults and to the coronary risk factors [29]. Obesity and the excess of adiposity are due to an imbalance between calories ingested and those spent. Environmental factors such as overfeeding or physical inactivity has been identified as the main causes of obesity in children [6,15].

In the last decades, diverse scientific studies have demonstrated that if physical exercise is practiced regularly it provides important health benefits [10,32,42,46,48]. The studies of adult populations suggest, generally, a protective relation between physical activity and the incidence of coronary diseases [21,40,50]. Physical inactivity is a predictor of coronary diseases, with a similar predictive power to the more traditional factors such as hypertension, hypercholesterolemia and tobacco addiction. Thus, according to Richardson et al. (2004) [50], the possibilities of a fatal cardiovascular disease fall progressively with the increase of energy expenditure. Twisk (2001) [60] affirms that 35% of the deaths by this type of diseases could be prevented with an adapted level of physical activity.

In summary, we could say that physical activity affects the following risk factors of cardiovascular disease by:

- Reducing the arterial pressure.
- Reducing the viscosity of the blood.
- Reducing the LDL-C levels and increasing those of HDL-C.
- Reducing the circulating catecholamine levels.
- Improving the healthy habits.

It is important to indicate that the lowering of the risk factors for cardiovascular diseases is only associated to those who maintain a certain level of continued physical activity throughout the life. For this reason, if the behaviour of children is more easily mouldable, it can be assumed that the daily activity habits formed during their childhood, will remain during their adult age [31,37,46]. This is the reason why it is believed to be more efficient to prioritize relevant education programs for children.

Tobacco consumption is the most important preventable cause of avoidable morbidity and mortality in the developed countries [5,45,54]. 500.000 deaths occur annually as a result of tobacco consumption in Europe and 40,000 in Spain. In addition more than 90% of the cases of lung cancer are attributed to tobacco. Chronic respiratory processes, associated to a great extent with tobacco consumption, are one of the main causes of labour incapacity and limited activity [45]. Tobacco consumption is also the most important modifiable risk factor for coronary disease. This risk increases with both a decrease in the age at which the tobacco consumption began and with an increase in the number of cigarettes consumed per day [41].

One of the most important problems with smokers regards their lifestyle and its repercussion on the quality of life. It is possible to distinguish the following two relevant points [16,22]:

(a) To smoke is a habit that does not appear separately but rather in association with other health risk factors. Generally smokers:

- Consume more alcohol and other drugs.
- Have a sedentary lifestyle.
- Their nutritional diets are less healthy.
- Generally consume more coffee and others stimulants.

(b) The second point relates to the sensation of a loss of control. When a smoker wishes to stop smoking and fails, frequently he feels that the tobacco "dominates him". This can end up with the sensation that they are unable to control their addiction; this sensation can also become general to other scopes of their life. To smoke is related to a lower level of self-control and search for immediate satisfaction; for this reason, addictive habits are more frequent in smokers and less frequent are those habits requiring long term reinforcement (for example, sport practice). The prevention of tobacco consumption in adolescents is not only important due to its effects on health, as this habit can act as an introduction to other drugs, the use and abuse of the alcohol and to the development of other injurious habits [16]. The scientific literature shows that smoking from an early age is associated with a great probability of smoking during adulthood and a smaller probability of stopping this habit in the future [42]. In recent years, health professionals have changed their emphasis from dealing with the adult smokers to preventing the consumption of tobacco in children. Almost all adult smokers began their habit during their adolescence, (i.e. before 15 years of age) [7] when tobacco consumption is a practice that is strongly affected by the individuals peers [16]. The aim of this work is to study in a representative sample of Madrilenian adolescents, the existing associations between markers of cardiovascular health such as blood pressure, body composition, tobacco consumption and the level of physical activity (LPA).

Material and Methods

Data were taken from different districts of Madrid including different types of education centres (public and private) with adolescents of different socio-economic levels. 35 education centres were randomly chosen, from 16 of the 21 districts of Madrid, comprising of 18 public and 17 private centres. In each centre subjects from 13 to 17 years were randomly selected.

2646 letters of consent were given to the parents of the adolescents. 1622 (61.3%) subjects returned written consent from which 578 were chosen randomly to participate in the study. From the 578 subjects 474 returned valid surveys, the final study population group was comprised of 204 boys (43%) and 270 girls (57%). According to that sample, considering the universe of the secondary students of the Municipality of Madrid during the academic course 2004-2005, it was obtained an error of ±6.9%, at the level of confidence of 95.5%. Table 1 shows the distribution of the subjects studied by ages and gender respectively. It should be noted that the sample is representative of the adolescents of Madrid.

Table 1. Distribution of the individuals in the sample by age and sex

			Sex		total
			boys	girls	
Age	13	N	21	28	49,
		Percentage	4,4%	5,9%	10,3%
	14	N	72	63	135
		Percentage	15,2%	13,3%	28,5%
	15	N	53	99	152
		Percentage	11,2%	20,9%	32,1%
	16	N	41	50	91
		Percentage	8,7%	10,6%	19,3%
	17	N	13	23	36
		Percentage	2,7%	4,9%	7,6%
	18	N	4	5	9
		Percentage	0,8%	1,0%	1,8%
	19	N	0	2	2
		Percentage	0,0%	0,4%	0,4%
Total		N	204	270	474
		Percentage	43%	57%	100%

After collecting a signed authorization of their parents or tutors, each participant was measured using anthropometric techniques, including the measurement of blood pressure. All the data were collected following a principle of total guarantee of the anonymity of the contributed data.

All the measurements were carried out by two graduate subjects, a man and a woman, with a degree in Physical Activity and Sports and properly trained for this task. Each one took the data to the subjects from his/her same gender.

In order to measure the LPA of the subjects of the sample, it was used the Modifiable Questionnaire of Physical Activity for Adolescentes [2] previously translated and validated for its use in Spain [16]. Considering the Longitudinal Amsterdam Growth And Health Study (ALGHS) [62] and following the recommendations of the English Health Education Authority (HEA) and the American College of Sport Medicine (ACSM), the following classification of the physical activity has been used:

- ≥49 METs/Week = Active/very active.
- 28-49 METs/ Week = Moderately active.
- <28 METs/ Week = Inactive/Sedentary.

Besides the questionnaire of physical activity, the general survey included questions about certain sociodemographic details. Two of the details were the type of educative centre of the adolescent and the educative level of the parents, variables that were used to determine the socioeconomic status (SES) of the adolescent. The questionnaire also included questions about the consumption habits including the tobacco consumption of both the adolescent as well as that of the people of their surroundings other questions regarded variables such as the weekly money availability.

With respect to the measurement of blood pressure, with the purpose of to avoid the slants of the observer, it was decided to use semiautomatic electronic devices (Omron 705CP) validated [20] according to the criteria of the American Asociation of Medical Instrument and of the British Hypertension Society. As definitive result were used the average of 2 valid readings of the blood pressure. According to the values of reference proposed for Spanish children and adolescents by the Spanish Cooperative Group for the Study of the Cardiovascular Risk Factors in Childhood and Adolescence in Spain [27]. To consider a subject as systolic and/or diastolic hypertensive the values that surpassed percentile 95 for their age and gender were used. In table 2 these values are exposed:

It should be noted that that all the subjects included in this work fulfilled the criteria of the WHO [28] regarding the standardization of the measurement of the blood pressure.

In order to calculate the subcutaneous fat, triceps, subscapular, suprailiac, abdominal, frontal thigh and medial leg skinfolds were measured with a Holtain calliper (Holtain Ltd, Dydef, UK), which is the recommended by the International Biological Programme [65].

For the calculation of the body fat percentaje, the Carter's equations were used [47]:

Boys: $\%BF = 0.1051 * \sum 6\text{Skinfolds} + 2.585$

Girls: $\%BF = 0.1548 * \sum 6\ \text{Skinfolds} + 3.580$

Table 2. Values of percentile 95 (en mmHg) of the blood pressure as a function of the age and the gender

Age (years)	Girls		*Boys*	
	Systolic BP	Diastolic BP	Systolic BP	*Diastolic BP*
12	133	80	134	*80*
13	135	80	139	*78*
14	133	80	138	*78*
15	135	80	145	*81*
16	134	81	147	*80*
17	137	80	152	*82*
18	*137*	*80*	*152*	*87*

Table 3. Classification of the subjects as a function of their level of body fat

CLASSIFICATION	BOYS	GIRLS
Thin	< 8%	< 13%
Optimum	8-15%	13-20%
Light overweight	16-20%	21-25%
Overweight	21-24%	25-32%
Obese	≥25%	≥33%

As can be observed in table 3, the classification of the subjects according to their level of body fat on the basis of the criteria of the Manual of Kinanthropometry of the Spanish Federation of Sport Medicine [47].

Concerning the compiled data processing, a datasheet in Microsoft Excel was designed. Those data were analyzed using the statistical program SPSS 11.5, concluding the study in September of 2005.

Firstly, a univariant analysis was carried out, in order to describe separately each variable. This analysis was complemented with the study of associations between variables. For this last one the chi-squared test of bivariant independence was applied, by simplicity, or test ANOVA, if the normality assumption were verified, working in each case at the confidence level of 95%.

Results

Physical Activity

For the whole sample, it was observed that 44.1% of the subjects have a high or very high LPA, 30.2% are moderately active while 25.7% are inactive or sedentary.

In addition, separating by gender and with the previously indicated classification, a substantial difference was found (χ^2=64.89; p=0.000) in the LPA of boys and girls, as showed in figure 1, where it can be seen that 64.7% of boys are active or very active whilst 35.6% of girls are inactive or sedentary.

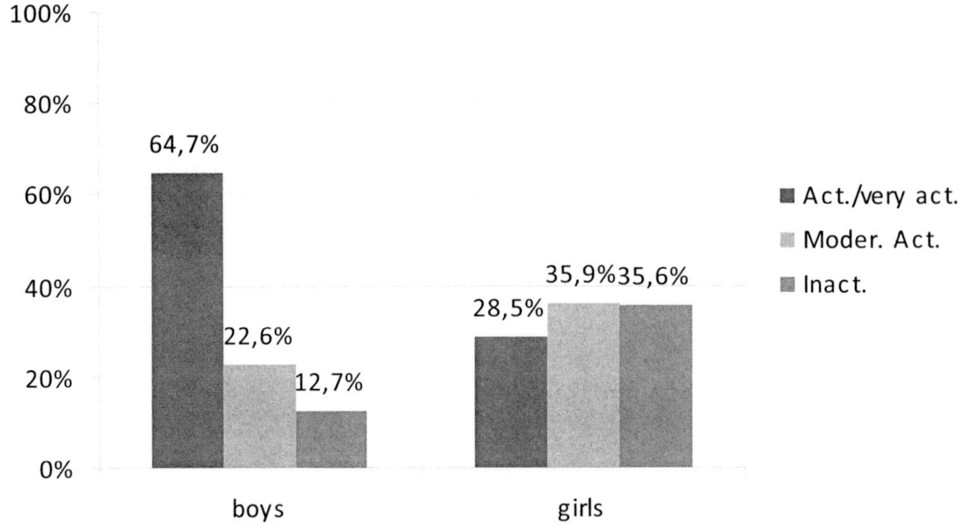

Figure 1. Distribution of the subjects in the sample by gender and physical activity level.

A significant relation has been found between the PAL of girls of the sample with the age (χ^2=27.25; p=0.007), but not for boys (χ^2=9.57; p=0.478). Furthermore, figure 2 reveals that the volume of physical activity decreased with age for girls.

Another significant relation (χ2=14.01; p=0.000) was found between the PAL and the SES in girls with the girls of the lower SES being more inactive and sedentary than the ones of the upper SES. Thus, 25.4% of the girls of the upper SES were inactive in comparison with 46.1% of the girls of the lower SES, this number rose to 50.9% for girls of age 16 or more years of the lower SES.

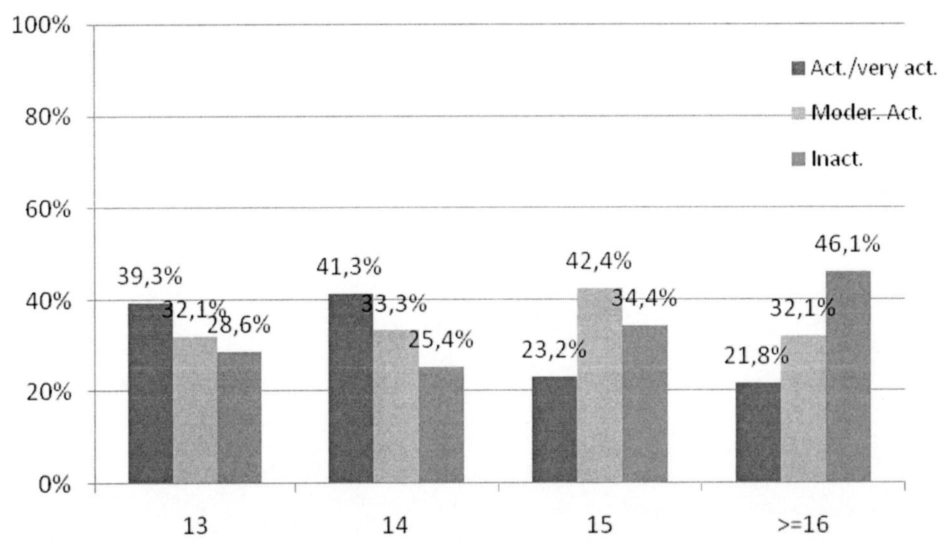

Figure 2. Distribution of girls in the sample by age and physical activity level.

Body Fat Level

With regard to the corporal adiposity level, a remarkable difference between boys and girls was detected (figure 3), which was checked by applying the ANOVA test ($F=556.79$; $p=0.000$). Average values, as a percentage of corporal adiposity, of 11.23 for boys and 20.36 for girls were found with the corresponding sample errors being of the order of 0.24 and 0.28 respectively. The classification of the subjects of the sample, according to that proposed by the Spanish Sport Medicine Federation [47], is summarized in table 4. We must indicate that these results may contain a certain bias because they do not include the data corresponding to 10 women who were obviously overweight and refused to be measured.

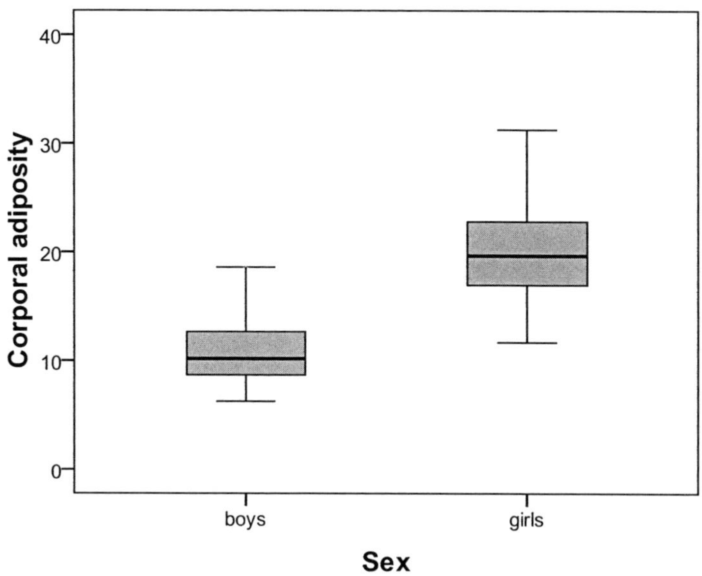

Figure 3. Box plot of percentage of body fat and gender.

Table 4. Relative levels of body weight as a function of the level of body fat in boys and girls of the sample

	All		Boys		Girls	
	N	%	N	%	N	%
Thin	25	5.3	20	9.8	5	1.9
Optimum	291	61.4	154	75.5	137	50.7
Light overweight	111	23.4	26	12.7	85	31.5
overweight	43	9.1	4	2	39	14.4
Obese	4	0.8	0	0	4	1.5
Total	474	100	204	100	270	100

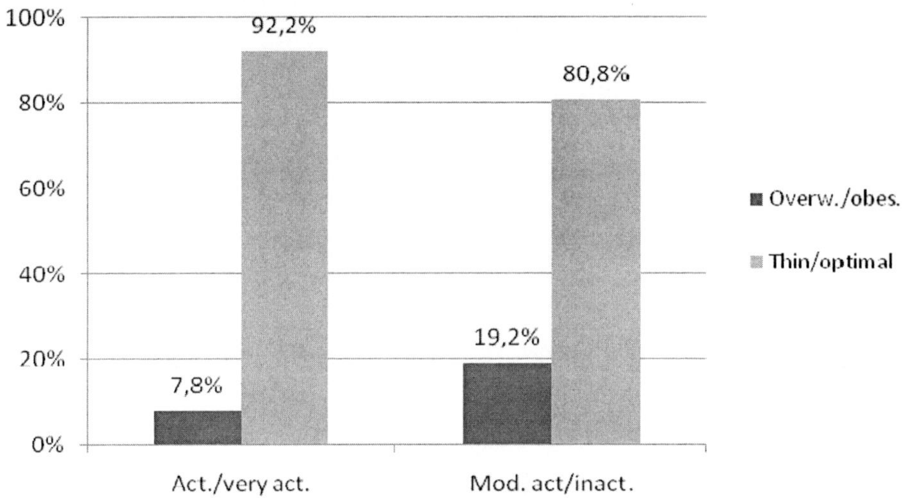

Figure 4. Distribution of the girls of the sample as a function of their level of physical activity and body fat.

On the basis of the above mentioned classification, a significant relation was found between the PAL and the body fat in girls ($\chi2$=24.49; p=0.002), but not in boys ($\chi2$=6.98; p=0.323). In the case of girls it can be observed in figure 4 that there exists important percentage differences regarding the increased tendency to be overweight when the individual's physical activity is at best moderate.

Tobacco Consumption

It was observed that:

- 35.8% of boys and 44.4% of girls tried smoking at least once in their life, but no significant relation (χ^2=4.52; p=0.104) was found between the gender and whether the individual had tried smoking at least once. Restricting our data to the subjects of 16 or more years we observed that 48.6% of boys of the upper SES and a 63.7% of girls of the lower had tried smoking at least once in their life.
- The tobacco consumption increase with the age (χ^2=59.95; p=0.000) in both girls and boys. The tobacco consumption increase strongly from the age 13 (6.1%), 14 (16.3%) until 48.6% at 16.
- The SES is also a significant variable for the tobacco consumption (χ^2=18.29; p=0.000). It was observed that the percentage of smokers is bigger among the subjects of the lower SES (50.2%) than those of the upper one (30.9%).
- Restricting our data to the subjects of 16 years or more, in the upper SES the smokers are balanced by gender (50% boys and 50% girls), whereas in the lower SES almost twice as many girls smoke as boys (34.9% of boys and 65.1% of girls).

Regarding the relation between the tobacco consumption and PAL, we observed an inverse significant relation for boys (χ^2=10.08; p= 0.039) but not for girls.

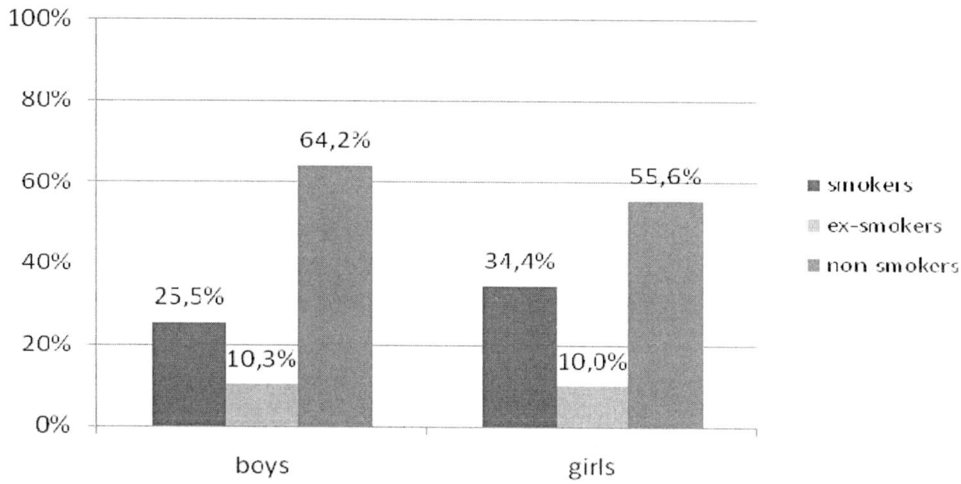

Figure 5. Distribution of the tobacco consumption of the subjects of the sample in the last year.

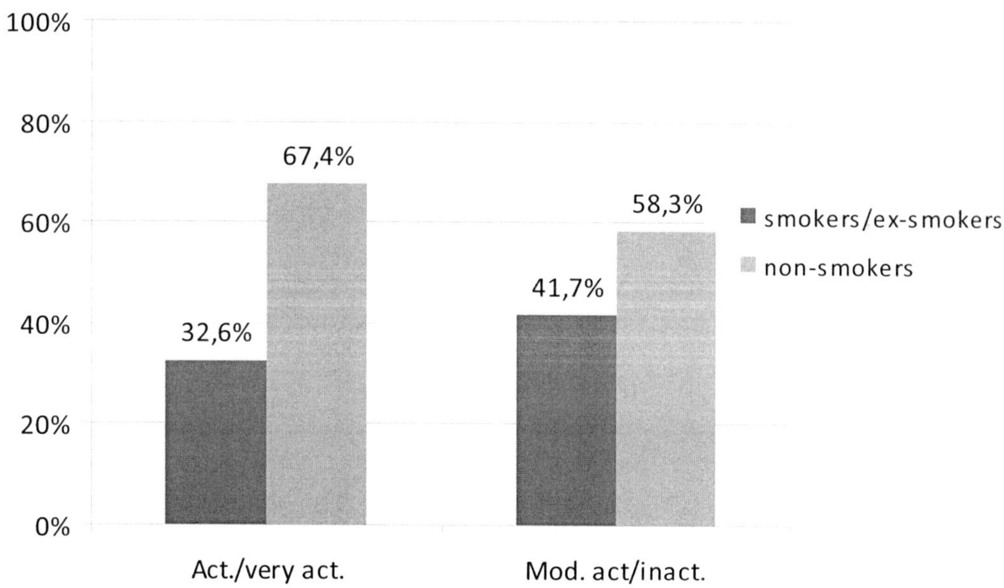

Figure 6. Distribution of men's level of physical activity by tobacco consumption.

We also found a very interesting relation between the weekly money availability and tobacco consumption (χ^2=40.34; p= 0.000) for both boys and girls. The more money is available for young people, the higher the tobacco consumption is.

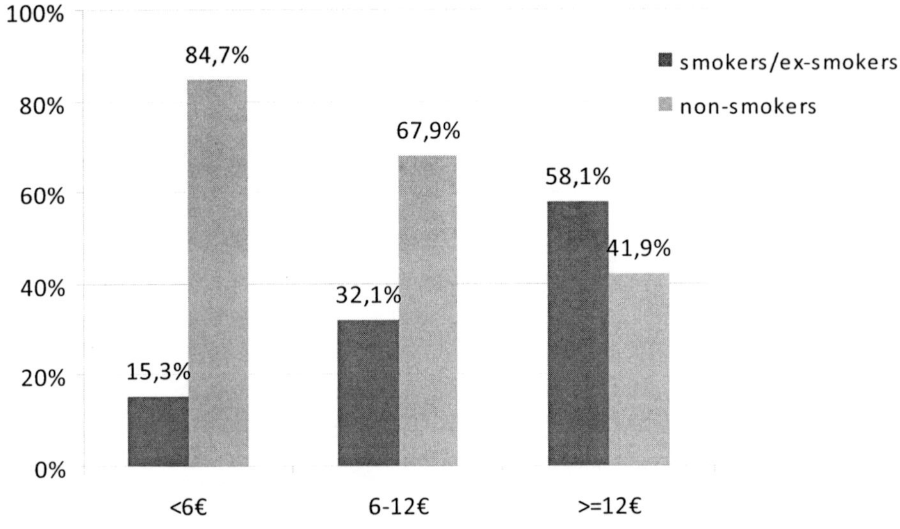

Figure 7. Distribution of the individuals in the sample by money availability and tobacco consumption.

Blood Pressure

The obtained data of the blood pressure (systolic and diastolic) are summarized in the figure 8.

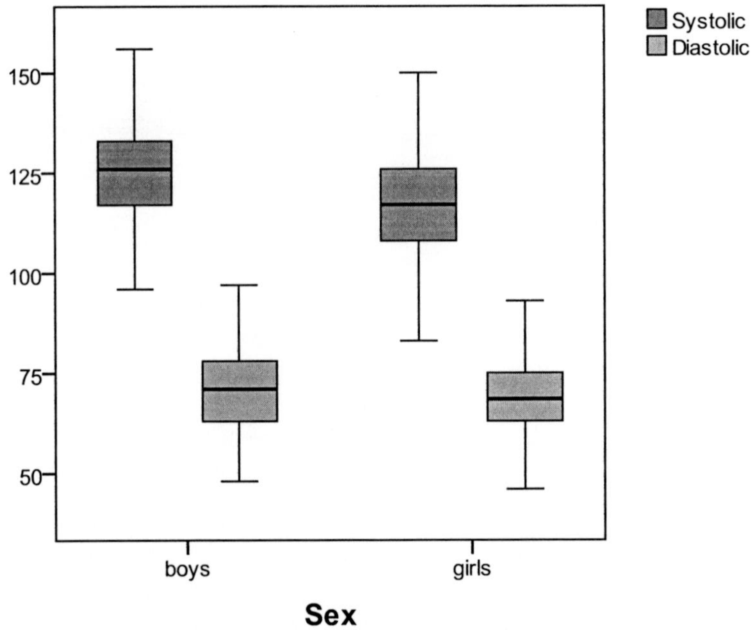

Figure 8. Box-plots of systolic blood pressure and diastolic blood pressure by gender.

We detected a significant relationship between gender and the systolic blood pressure ($F=36.48$; $p=0.000$), where the girls had the lowest levels and less dispersed data. The results for the diastolic blood pressure were non significant ($F=3.59$; $p=0.058$). In fact, we found average values of the systolic/diastolic blood pressure of 125.6/71.3 mmHg for boys and 118/69.4 mmHg for girls respectively. Sampling errors of 0.95/0.78 mmHg and 0.83/0.67 mmHg were respectively obtained for boys and for girls.

In addition, it was observed that 11.5% of girls and 11.8% of boys of the sample had systolic hypertension and 4.4% of girls and 9.8% of boys had diastolic hypertension. The subjects with both systolic and diastolic hypertension amounted to 2.2% of the girls and 1.5% of the boys.

With respect to the relation between the PAL and the blood pressure, the ANOVA test only found a relation for the diastolic Blood pressure and PAL in boys ($F=5.41$; $p=0,021$). 95% confidence intervals of the order of 67.9-72 mmHg for the diastolic blood pressure in the active or very active adolescents or of 71.2-76.9 mmHg in the other cases were observed

In order to analyze the possible relations with other variables in which the normality hypothesis was not verified, the chi-square test of independence was used and the data of both pressures have been grouped in 6 intervals as follows:

Interval	1	2	3	4	5	6
Systolic BP	Until 105	105-115	115-125	125-135	135-145	More than 145
Diastolic BP	Until 60	60-65	65-70	70-75	75-80	More than 80

With these results, it is possible to observe that the relation between tobacco consumption and the systolic blood pressure ($\chi2=2.64$; $p= 0.989$) or diastolic blood pressure ($\chi2=10.85$; $p= 0.369$) does not exist, neither for boys nor for girls. The same happens if we analyze the existence of an association for the level of body fat with the systolic blood pressure ($\chi2=13.26$; $p= 0.866$) or with diastolic blood pressure ($\chi2=20.85$; $p= 0.405$).

Discusion and Conclusion

The results of our study were obtained exclusively with students of the Municipality of Madrid. However, we believe these results can be extended to the adolescents of Madrid in general, if the number of subjects in the study and the way in which the sampling was done is taken into account. It should be noted that methodological limitations exist for this type of study due to the lack of objectivity in the measurement of the LPA. The majority of authors however consider the use of questionnaires for adolescents and adults acceptable because they enable one to study these populations [25,46].

It noted that there exists a shortage of studies on Spanish adolescents with a sample similar to that we obtained and used in this investigation, this has caused us in some cases to make comparisons with international studies. In our study one of the most remarkable observations is that for our sample of adolescents of the Municipality of Madrid, 25.7% have a LPA lower than the recommended. Even so, these results are not as worrisome as those obtained in a sample of a 367 adolescents of Teruel [13,14], a Spanish city of medium size located in more rural surroundings. We can see the comparison of both studies summarized in table 5.

Table 5. Summary of the results on the level of physical activity get in our work compared with the one of Cantera and Devís (2000)

STUDY	Boys			*Girls*		
	Active and Very Active	Mod. Active	Inactive and Sedentary	Active and Very Active	Mod. Active	*Inactive and Sedentary*
Teruel 1997	45.2%	23.4%	30.3%	21.2%	24%	*50.3%*
Madrid 2005	*64.7%*	*22.6%*	*12.7%*	*28.5%*	*35.9%*	*35.6%*

We also got better results than the found those presented by Tercedor et al. (2007) for adolescents from different parts of Spain (40.8% of inactive subjects), Pate, Heath, Dowda and Trost (1996) on a representative sample of North American adolescents of whom 14.1% were sedentary and 22.8% were very active, Savage and Scott (1998) on North American adolescents from the countryside (32% of active adolescents and 33.2% of inactive or sedentary) or in the results obtained by Van Mechelen et al. (2000) in the ALGHS (32.8% of inactive subjects).

On the other hand, the results of the present work are not as optimistic as mentioned in the review by Aaron and Laporte (1997) of the "Youth Risk Behavior Survey", the "National Children and Youth Survey" and the "Adolescent Injury Study Control", which indicate that only 10.4% of the adolescents are inactive compared to 63.7% active subjects.

We can affirm that our results are equal to the average found in the bibliography. Nevertheless the fact that 25.7%, of the subjects were inactive or sedentary in our sample is a worrisome value in these ages due to the repercussions that this can have in the medium and long term future on the individual's health. This is even more so when we consider that, after adolescence the LPA tends to fall strongly for both boys and girls [39]. In fact in our sample, as in other works [57], a significant fall in the physical activity of the girls with the age is observed. Another point to emphasize is that the diversity in the methodology used to measure the LPA and to classify the subjects makes it difficult to compare studies. For this reason, we propose that it is of vital importance to unify the criteria used by different researcher on physical activity and its determinants.

Concerning the behavior of the physical activity with the age, our results with respect to the boys are different to the majority of the reviewed studies that indicate that the physical activity falls with the age [10,51,59-61]. Our results agree partially with Aaron et al. (1993) that did not find relation between the level of physical activity and age between boys, and totally with Cantera and Devís (2000 and 2002) in a study carried out in Teruel (Spain). Therefore we believe it is necessary to examine in detail this relation in future studies, to determine if our results are due to a particular characteristic of our sample, or if they are due to something commonly found in Spanish adolescents. Another thing that is necessary to examine is the effect of the fact that the majority of the boys in our sample (81.4%) are between 14 and 16 years old, this corresponds to the stage immediately subsequent to peak growth. According to Vanden Eynde, Germ, Vienna, Vuylsteke-Auters and Ghesquiere (1989), this is the moment of greatest physical activity during ones life.

As in the great majority of reviewed studies, we found very clear differences in the LPA between genders [4,10,14,25,35,51,57,62,66]. Nevertheless, our results for girls, although very worrisome, are not as dramatic as those found amongst Italian girls of 14 to18 years where only 8% were active and 65% were inactive or sedentary [12].

Another common result that we found is the relation between the LPA and the SES among girls. It can be observed in our sample that girls of the upper SES are mostly at least moderately active whereas the majority of girls of the lower SES are inactive or sedentary. These results agree totally with the ones of Aaron et al. (1993) but it should be noted that most of the reviewed literature [4,42,59] show a significant relation between these variables, with the subjects of the upper SES always the more actives.

Due to all these results and the comparison with the reviewed literature, we suggested that campaigns for the promotion of physical activity and sport could be necessary for the general population and specifically for feminine population of the lower SES.

As we already commented previously, it is especially interesting to compare our results with the ALGHS [62], since they used the same criteria to classify the LPA of the adolescents. Average values of the LPA obtained in this study with subjects among 13 and 16 years can be observed in the table 6. An important point to remember is that this data were taken in 1981. We can observe in table 4, the very interesting comparison of our data with the "European Youth Heart Study" [10], since their data were collected with objectives methods in 2001 in subjects of 15 years from four European countries: Denmark, Portugal, Estonia and Norway.

We observe a great similarity in the three works with respect to the LPA of girls, whereas it seems that the current European boys are clearly more active than they were in the Netherlands in 1981.

Regarding the found significant difference between gender and the level of body fat, our results agree with all similar studies [59], In the case of girls it is observed that as the adiposity level is increased then the level of physical activity is clearly reduced. In fact the majority of the thin girls are, at least, active whereas this trend changes amongst the overweight or obese girls.

Table 6. Comparison of the results of the physical activity level of Dutch (1983), European (2001) and Madrilenian (2005). It should be noted that the subjects with moderate physical activity were considered active

STUDY	Boys		*Girls*	
	Active	Inactive	Active	*Inactive*
The Netherland 1981	69.35%	30.65%	64.05%	*35.95%*
Europe 2001	81.9%	18.1%	62%	*38%*
Madrid 2005	*87.3%*	*12.7%*	*64.4%*	*35.6%*

Amongst boys, the differences are less clear, as there were no observed differences between the LPA for "thin" to "light overweight"; nevertheless, when the subject is overweight it is observed that there exits a preference to be inactive or sedentary.

Our results agree totally with those of Boreham, Twisk and Savage (1997) and only partially, since they also find this association between boys, with those obtained by Raitakari et al. (1997).

According to Aaron and Laporte (1997), although some cross-sectional studies have found an inverse relation between physical activity and the measures of skin folds, others have not found this association. Nevertheless, even though a relation was observed, it was not possible to determine its direction. Little physical activity leads to obesity or the obese practice less physical activity? This question only can be answered by a longitudinal study. Nevertheless, according to the same authors, an exercise program will diminish the body fat level in obese adolescents. In fact, in our study, there is an evident parallel with age in girls between the evolution of the body fat and the level of physical activity: as the age increases, the physical activity levels lower and body fat levels increase.

Although overweight and obesity can be due to genetic and/or metabolic causes, this is like to account for very few cases [59]. Overweight and obesity are mainly caused by an incorrect energy balance, produced by a high nutritional ingestion that is not compensated with sufficient energy expenditure due to a deficit of physical activity.

The prevalence of overweight and obesity are increasing in such an alarming way in the western countries that some studies already speak of this phenomenon in terms of epidemia [9,64]. We must always consider the consequences of the loss of physical activity in daily life, its effect on the prevalence of overweight and obese people and the effect that this has on the economy of the countries that suffer this way of life, and also the consequential strong rates of premature morbidity and mortality. For example, in the U.S.A., the direct cost generated by inactivity and obesity consumes 9.4% of the annual medical cost [29], whereas in Spain, this number is up to around 7% [64] already.

Although the studies that analyze the association between body fat and the LPA in adults obtain conclusive results, usually this does not happen in the studies of adolescents. It seems that, in many cases, amongst young subjects there has not yet been time for the effects of physical inactivity to be observed in their corporal composition.

Besides improving the level of physical activity, see also De Vito, Latorre, Langiano, Berardi and Ricciardi (1999), we think that the nutritional education is another basic question from a preventive point of view. Many of the errors that take place in relation to nutrition are related with a lack of information and, mainly, with a lack of understanding.

With respect to the tobacco consumption, the increase in its consumption with age for adolescents is a common finding in both Spanish and international ones [7,18]. The prevalence of tobacco consumption amongst the boys and girls of our sample is equivalent to the average observed in the reviewed national studies for subjects of similar ages [57].

As we can observe in table 7, it seems that in all the studies of Spanish adolescents in the last 15 years there exists a greater prevalence of tobacco consumption for girls than for boys. All the studies however do not observe significant differences. In any case, if we compare the results of different studies carried out with adolescents with others carried out with adults

[58] for whom historically men were bigger smokers [17], we observed a certain feminization of the adolescent tobacco consumption.

Table 7. Comparison of tobacco consumption in different Spanish studies

AUTHORS	PLACE	YEAR	*AGES*	N	BOYS SMOKERS	GIRLS SMOKERS
Palau et al.	Navarra	1993	14-17	910	15,7%	16,2%
Sánchez	Madrid	1996	Secund.	1.360	19,5%	38%
C.A.M.	Madrid	1997	13-16	-	36,7%	40%
Cordente	Madrid	2005	13-17	474	25,5%	34,4%
Tercedor et al.	Spain	2007	12-19	1.300	21,5%	24,5%

We found an inverse association between tobacco consumption and LPA in boys. Thus, the smokers present the greater percentage of inactivity or sedentary behavior, the ex-smokers tend to be at least moderately active whereas those that never smoked were active or very active. Our results are similar to those found in Finland [55], in Barcelona (Spain) [38] and they only agree partially with those obtained by Tercedor et al. (2007) in a sample of adolescents of different parts of Spain. On the other hand, our results are opposed to those found in the U.S.A.[1,4] where was founded a significant relation between tobacco consumption and the LPA for girls but not for boys.

In the literature, generally associations between LPA and tobacco consumption in children do not exist. Nevertheless, between adolescents one begins to observe a certain relation, either between boys or between girls or even in both. Finally, between adults the association between both variables appears very clear. Therefore it is possible to think that the age is an important factor for observing this type of associations.

As we already commented in the introduction of this work, the adolescent tobacco consumption (and also the one of other legal and illegal drugs) is framed essentially in the relation with the peers due to a question of behaving the same and personal experimentation. It seems necessary to take initiatives that allows the adolescents to try themselves in other scopes that are not related to drug consumption. We guess that sport can be one of those alternatives, since is intimately related to self-overcoming necessity. Unfortunately, in spite of some initiatives which have achieved great success, in Spain they are scarce public sport facilities that can essentially be used for 24 hours of the day, and during the weekend when the consumption of drugs is greatest.

An interesting association that we found is the one existing between the tobacco consumption and the money availability in adolescents. This result is even more interesting if we take into account the agreement in all the works that have treated these variables [7,34]. Thus, we can confirm that with an increase in the money in the pocket of adolescents the consumption of legal and illegal drug could become more a norm than an exception. For this reason we propose that it is highly necessary to inform parents about the danger for their children's health if they have too much money and to act before the child reaches 15 years old. As according to Ariza and Nebot (2002) it is less probable to begin to smoke in adulthood if the individual did not start young. We already commented in the introduction on this work regarding the adolescent tobacco consumption and how it is essentially framed in the relation with the peers. It is therefore possible to assume that with little money in their pockets, adolescents will channel their experimentation tendencies towards others healthier activities.

Table 8. Comparison of the results of the blood pressure (in mmHg) obtained in different international studies

AUTHORS	Country	YEAR	AGE	Blood Pressure BOYS	*Blood Pressure GIRLS*
Paulus et al.	Belgium	1999	12-17	125/74	*122/74*
V. Mechelen et al.	Holland	2000	13-16	126.6/76.1	*122,1/73,2*
Twisk et al.*	Holland	2002	32	135/86	*125/83*
Boreham et al.	Ireland	2002	12-15	118,5/76	*107.5/71,5*
Cordente et al.	*Madrid (Spain)*	*2003*	*13-17*	*125.6/71,3*	*118/69.4*

(*) The study of Twisk et al. (2002) is a longitudinal continuation of the study of Van Mechelen et al. (2000).

We can add that our results agree partially with those studies that do not find a relation between LPA and blood pressure in either gender [19,48].

Concerning blood pressure, we can see in table 8, a comparison of our study with the found average values in the different reviewed works. Regarding the observed rate of systolic and diastolic hypertension (2.2% of girls and 1.9% of boys), our results are inferiors to the 11.4% found in a sample of Belgium [44] subjects with similar characteristics to ours. We agree with Soler, Gil and Rey (1992) regarding the prevalence of systolic hypertension being greater than diastolic (11.6% and 6.8% of the subjects respectively).

We did not find any relation for the blood pressure neither with body fat nor with consumption of tobacco. The absence of relations between blood pressure and the rest of treated variables (LPA, body fat and tobacco consumption) would support the idea that we already defended in the cases of the body composition and tobacco consumption with respect to the LPA. The effects of certain habits on the cardiovascular risk factors needs a longer time to be obvious. Therefore, it seems to be sensible to suggest new studies of the existing associations between these variables within the framework a longitudinal study. This would allow us to know exactly to what extent and in which moment the changes in each variable are obvious and to contribute, more efficiently to preventive solutions for preventing the appearance of health risk factors.

References

[1] Aaron, DJ; Dearwater, SR; Anderson, R; Olsen, T; Kriska, AM; Laporte, RE. Physical activity and the initiation of high-risk health behaviors in adolescents. *Medicine and Science in Sports and Exercise,* 1995; 27, 1639-1645.

[2] Aaron, DJ; Kriska, AM. Modifiable activity questionnaire for adolescents. *Med. Sci. Sports Exerc.* 1997; 29 (1 Supl 2): 79-82.

[3] Aaron, DJ; Kriska, AM; Dearwater, SR; Anderson, RL; Olsen, TL; Cauley, JA; Laporte, RE. The epidemiology of leisure physical activity in an adolescent population. *Medicine and Science in Sports and Exercise*, 1993; 25, 847-853.

[4] Aaron, DJ; Laporte, RE. Physical activity, adolescence and health: an epidemiological perspective. *Exerc. Sport Sci. Rev.* 1997; 25: 391-405.

[5] Abernathy, TJ; Massad, L; Romano-Dwyer, L. The relationship between smoking and self- esteem. *Adolescence,* 1995; 30, 899-907.

[6] Albright, AL; Stern, JS. Adipose tissue. Encyclopedia of Sports Medicine and Science. Internet Society for Sport Science (1998, may). Available in: Http://www.sportsci.org.

[7] Ariza, C; Nebot, M. Predictores de la iniciación al consumo de tabaco en escolares de enseñanza secundaria de Barcelona y Lleida. *Revista Española de Salud Pública*, 2002; 76, 227-238.

[8] Badía, X; Rovira, J; Tresseras, R; Trinxet, C; Segú JL. El coste de la hipertensión en España. *Medicina Clínica*, 1992; 99, 769-773.

[9] Banegas, JR. Epidemiología de la hipertensión arterial en España. Situación actual y perspectivas. *Hipertensión.* 2005; 22: 353-62.

[10] Boreham, C; Twisk, J; Neville, C; Savage, M; Murray, L; Gallagher, A. Associations between physical fitness and cardiovascular risk factors in young adulthood: the Northern Ireland young hearts project. *Int. J. Sports Med.* 2002; 23 [1 supplement 2]: 22-6.

[11] Boreham, CA; Twisk, J; Savage, MJ. Physical activity, sports participation, and risk factors in adolescents. *Med. Sci. Sports Exerc.* 1997; 29: 788-93.

[12] Cale, L; Almond, L Physical activity levels of secondary-aged children: a review. *Health Educ. J.* 1992; 51: 192-7.

[13] Cantera, MA; Devís J. Physical activity levels of secondary school spanish adolescents. Eur J Physical Educ. 2002; 5: 28-44.

[14] Cantera, MA; Devís, J. La promoción de la actividad física relacionada con la salud en el ámbito escolar. Implicaciones y propuestas a partir de un estudio realizado entre adolescentes. *Apunts.* 2000; 6: 54-62.

[15] Caspersen, CJ; Nixon, PA; Durant, RH. Physical activity epidemiology applied to children and adolescent. *Exercise and Sport Science Reviews*, 1998; 26, 241-403.

[16] Cordente Martínez, CA. Estudio epidemiológico del nivel de actividad física y de otros parámetros de interés relacionados con la salud bio-psico-social de los alumnos de E.S.O. del Municipio de Madrid [Doctoral dissertation]. Toledo: Universidad de Castilla-La Mancha [2006-12-12]. Available from: http://www.cafyd.com/tesis12cordente.pdf.

[17] De Bourdeuaudhuij, I; Van Oost, P. A cluster-analytical approach toward physical activity and other health related behavior. *Medicine and Science in Sports and Exercise*, 1999; 31, 605-612.

[18] De Vito, E; La Torre, G; Langiano, E; Berardi, D; Ricciardi, G. Overweight and obesity among secondary school children in central Italy. *Eur. J. Epidemiol.* 1999; 15: 649-54.

[19] Dencker, M; Thorsson, O; Karlsson, MK; Linden, C; Svensson, J; Wollmer, P; Andersen, LB. Daily physical activity in Swedish children aged 8-11 years. *Scand. J. Med. Sci. Sports*. 2006; 16: 252-7.

[20] Divisón Garrote, JA. Medidas de presión arterial de forma semiautomática en el diagnostico de la hipertensión arterial. Comparación con otros métodos diagnósticos y estudio de su variabilidad y reproducibilidad [Tesis Doctoral]. Madrid: Universidad Autónoma de Madrid; 1998.

[21] Ferriéres J. Facteurs de risque, lipoproteines et activité physique et sportive. *Science et Sports*, 2004; 19 (3), 118-123.

[22] Froján, MX; Santacreu, J. Uso de tabaco y otros hábitos de vida en estudiantes de la universidad autónoma de Madrid. *Adicciones*, 1992; 4 (2), 93-109.

[23] García del Pozo, J; Ramos Sevillano E; De Abajo, FJ; Mateos Campos, R. Utilización de antihipertensivos en España (1995-2001). *Rev. Esp. Cardiol.* 2004; 57: 241-9.

[24] García Ruiz, AJ; García Ruiz I, Aranda Lara, P; Montesinos, AC; Martos Crespo F; Sánchez De La Cuesta, F. Estudios sobre los Enfermos Hipertensos en Tratamientos en España durante el Periodo 1990-1993. *Revista Española De Salud Publica*, 1997; 71, 9-17.

[25] Gavarry, O ; Falgairette, G. L'activité physique habituelle au cours du développement. *Revue Canadienne de Physiologie Appliquée*, 2004; 29, 201-214.

[26] Grundy, SM; Blackburn, G; Higgins, M; Lauer, R; Perri, MG; Ryan, D. Physical activity in the prevention and treatment of obesity and its comorbidities: evidence report of independent panel to assess the role of physical activity in the treatment of obesity and its comorbidities. *Med. Sci. Sports Exerc.* 1999; 31: 1493-500.

[27] Grupo Cooperativo Español para el Estudio de los Factores de Riesgo Cardiovascular en la Infancia y Adolescencia. Factores de riesgo cardiovascular en la infancia y adolescencia en España. Estudio RICARDIN II: Valores de referencia. *An. Esp. Pediatr.* 1995; 43: 11-17.

[28] Guidelines Subcommittee.1999 World Health Organization-International society of hypertension guidelines for the management of the hypertension. *J. Hypertens.* 1999; 17: 151-83.

[29] Guo, SS; Chumlea, WC. Tracking of body mass index in children in relation to overweight in adulthood. *Am. J. Clin. Nutr.* 1999; 70: S145-8.

[30] Instituto Nacional de Estadística. Anuario Estadístico de España; 2001. Madrid: I.N.E.; 2001

[31] Janz, KF; Dawson, JD; Mahoney, LT. Tracking physical fitness and physical activity from childhood to adolescence: the Muscatine study. *Med Sci Sports Exerc.* 2000; 32: 1250-7.

[32] Krekoukia, M; Nassis, GP; Psarra, G; Skenderi, K; Chrousos, GP; Sidossis, LS. Elevated total and central adiposity and low physical activity are associated with insulin resistance in children. *Metabolism.* 2007; 56: 206-13.

[33] López Calbet, A; Dorado, C; Chavarren, J. Evaluación de la composición corporal mediante absorciometría fotónica dual de rayos X. In: Consejo Superior de Deportes, Editor. Métodos de Estudio de Composición Corporal en Deportistas. Madrid: Ministerio de Educación y Cultura. *Consejo Superior de Deportes*; 1996; 55-79.

[34] Martínez Álvarez, J; García González, J; Domingo Gutiérrez, M; Machín Fernández, AJ. Consumo de alcohol, tabaco y drogas en adolescentes. *Atención Primaria*, 1996; 18, 383-385.

[35] Michaud-Tomson, L; Davidson, M; Cuddihy, TF. Walk to school does it make a difference in children's physical activity levels? *ACHPER Healthy Lifestyles Journal*, 2004; 50 (3-4), 16-24.

[36] Morrow, JR; Krzsewinski-Malone, JA; Jackson, AW; Bungum, T J; Fitzgerald SJ. American adult's knowledge of exercise recommendations. *Research Quarterly for Exercises and Sport*, 2004; 75, 231-237.

[37] National Center for Chronic Disease Prevention and Health Promotion; Centers for Disease Control and Prevention. Guidelines for school and community programs to promote lifelong physical activity among young people. *J. Sch. Health*. 1997; 67: 202-19.

[38] Nebot, M; Comín, E; Villalbí, JR; Murillo, C. La actividad física de los escolares: un estudio transversal. *Revista de Sanidad e Higiene Pública*, 1991; 65, 325-331.

[39] Nelson, MC; Neumark-Stzainer, D; Hannan, PJ; Sirard, JR; Story, M Longitudinal and secular trends in physical activity and sedentary behavior during adolescence. *Pediatrics*. 2006; 118: 1627-34.

[40] Oja, P. (1995). Descriptive epidemiology of health-related physical activity and fitness. *Research Quarterly for Exercise and Sport*, 66, 303-312.

[41] Palau Bondíal, J; Reparaz Abaitual, F; Elcarte López, R; Iñigo Martínez, J; Ferreiro Mazón, H; Aldaz Izurzu, Y; Villa Elízagal, I. Distribución de las variables lipídicas en adolescentes fumadores. *Anales Españoles de Pediatría*, 1997; 46, 245-251.

[42] Pate, RR; Heath, GW; Dowda, M; Trost, SG. Associations between physical activity and other health behaviors in a representative sample of U.S. adolescents. *Am. J. Public Health*. 1996; 86: 1577-581.

[43] Pate, RR; Pfeiffer, KA; Trost, SG; Ziegler, P; Dowda M. Physical Activity among children attending preschools. *Pediatrics*. 2004; 114: 1258-63.

[44] Paulus, D; Saint-Remy, A; Jeanjean, M. Blood pressure during adolescence: a study among belgian adolescents selected from a high cardiovascular risk population. *Eur. J. Epidemiol.* 1999; 15: 783-90

[45] Pérez Ollé, R; Pérez Ollé, J. Prevalencia del consumo de tabaco y alcohol, actitudes y creencias en estudiantes de bachillerato de la provincia de Tarragona (España). *Anales Españoles de Pediatría*, 1996; 45, 583-590.

[46] Perula de Torres, LA; Lluch, C; Ruiz Moral, R; Espejo Espejo, J; Tapia, G; Mengual Luque, P. Prevalencia de actividad física y su relación con variables sociodemográficas y ciertos estilos de vida en escolares cordobeses. *Rev. Esp. Salud. Publica*. 1998; 72: 233-44.

[47] Porta, J; Galiano, D; Tejedo, A; González, JM. Valoración de la composición corporal. utopías y realidades. In: Esparza Ros F, Editor. Manual de Cineantropometría. Monografías FEMEDE. Madrid: *FEMEDE* 1993; 113-170.

[48] Raitakari, OT; Taimela, S; Porkka, KVK; Telama, R; Välimäki, I; Akerblom, HK; Viikari, JSA. Associations between physical activity and risk factors for coronary heart

disease: the cardiovascular risk in young finns study. *Med. Sci. Sports Exerc.* 1997; 29: 1055-61.

[49] Rhea, DJ. Physical activity and body image of female adolescents. *Journal of Physical Education, Recreation and Dance,* 1998; 69 (5), 27-31.

[50] Richardson, CR; Kriska, AM; Lantz, PM; Hayward, RA. Physical activity and mortality across cardiovascular disease risk groups. *Medicine and Science in Sports and Exercise*, 2004; 36, 1923-1929.

[51] Riddoch, CJ; Andersen, LB; Wedderkopp, N; Harro, M; Klasson-Heggebo, L; Sardinha, LB; Cooper, AR; Ekelund, U. Physical activity levels patterns of 9- and 15-years-old european children. *Med. Sci. Sports Exerc.* 2004; 36: 86-92.

[52] Savage, MP; Scott, LB. Physical activity and rural middle school adolescents. *J. Youth Adolesc.* 1998; 27: 245-253.

[53] Schmidt, GJ; Walkuski, JJ; Stensel, DJ. Estudio acerca de los factores de riesgo de enfermedades coronarias y actividad física en la juventud de Singapur. *Medicine and Science in Sport and Exercise,* 1998; 30, 105-113.

[54] Silber, TJ. Enfoque clínico de la atención de salud del adolescente. In Silbert TJ, Munist MM, Maddaleno M, Suárez Ojeda EN Editors, Manual de Medicina de la Adolescencia. Washington D. C.; *Organización Panamericana de la Salud*; 1992; 1-2.

[55] Simonen, R; Levälahti, E; Kaprio, J; Videman, T; Battié, MC. Multivariate genetic analysis of lifetime exercise an environmental factors. *Medicine and Science in Sports and Exercise*, 2004; 36, 1559-1566.

[56] Soler, MB; Gil, A; Rey, J. Estudio epidemiológico de la tensión arterial en una población escolar. *Aten Primaria.* 1992; 9: 212-4.

[57] Tercedor, P; Martín-Matillas, M; Chillón, P; Pérez López, IJ; Ortega, FB; Wärnberg, J; Ruiz, JR; Delgado, M; Grupo AVENA. Incremento del consumo de tabaco y disminución del nivel de práctica de actividad física en adolescentes españoles. Estudio AVENA. *Nutr Hosp.* 2007; 22(1):89-94.

[58] Tormo Díaz, MJ; Navarro Sánchez, C; Chirlaque López, MD; Pérez Flores, D. Factores de riesgo cardiovascular en la región de Murcia. *Revista Española de Salud Pública,* 1997; 71, 515-529.

[59] Tudor-Locke, C; Myers, AM. Challenges and opportunities for measuring physical activity in sedentary adults. *Sports Med.* 2001; 31: 91-100.

[60] Twisk, JWR. Physical activity for children and adolescents. *Sports Medicine*, 2001; 31, 617-627.

[61] Twisk, JWR; Kemper, HCG; Van Mechelen, W. Tracking of activity and fitness and the relationship with cardiovascular disease risk factors. *Medicine and Science in Sports and Exercise,* 2000; 32, 1455–1461.

[62] Van Mechelen, W; Twisk, JWR; Berheke Post, G; Snel, J; Kemper, HCG. Physical activity of young people: the Amsterdam longitudinal growth and health study. *Med. Sci. Sports Exerc.* 2000; 32: 1610-17.

[63] Vanden Eynde, B; Van Gerven, D; Vienne, D; Vuylsteke-Wauters, M; Ghesquier, J. Endurance fitness and peak height velocity in belgian boys. In Oseid S, Carlsen K Editors. Children And Exercise XIII. Champaign, Illinois: *Human Kinetics Publishers,* Inc.; , 1989; 19-27.

[64] Vázquez Sánchez, R; López Alemany, JM. Los costes económicos de la obesidad alcanzan el 7% del gasto sanitario [cited 2007-05-30]. Available from: http://www.economiadelasalud.com/Ediciones/03/PDF/03Analisis_Costes.pdf.

[65] Weiner, JS; Lourie, JA. Human biological. A guide to field methods. International Biological Programme (handbook nº 9). Oxford: Blackwell scientific; 1969.

[66] Welk, GJ; Schaben, JA; Shelley, M. Physical activity and physical fitness in children schooled at home and children attending public schools. *Pediatr. Exerc. Sci.* 2004; 16: 310-23.

In: Hypertension, Heredity and Stroke
Editor: Cristina Moratinos and Bruno Cardenas

ISBN 978-1-60741-496-4

Chapter 4

Ambulatory Blood Pressure Monitoring in Children with Glomerular Kidney Disease

Piotr Skrzypczyk, Małgorzata Panczyk-Tomaszewska, Iwona Bieroza and Maria Roszkowska-Blaim*
Department of Pediatrics and Nephrology, Medical University of Warsaw, Warsaw

Abstract

INTRODUCTION: Arterial hypertension and cardiovascular complications are common problems in patients with glomerulonephritis. Ambulatory blood pressure monitoring (ABPM) is a useful method for early evaluation of hypertension.

PURPOSE OF THE STUDY: The purpose of the study was to analyze ABPM parameters and to evaluate its usefulness in the evaluation of arterial hypertension in children with glomerular kidney disease.

MATERIAL AND METHODS: The study involved 47 children aged 4.5 to 18 (mean 14.2+3.3) years, including 17 patients with IgA nephropathy or Schoenlein-Henoch syndrome, 9 with idiopathic nephrotic syndrome, and 22 with other forms of glomerulonephritis. ABPM was performed in all children. The following ABPM parameters were analyzed: systolic, diastolic and mean blood pressure during 24 hrs (sBP/24h, dBP/24h, MAP/24h), activity (sBP/a, dBP/a, MAP/a) and resting period (sBP/r, dBP/r, MAP/r); systolic and diastolic blood pressure load during 24 hrs (sBPL/24h, dBPL/24h), activity (sBPL/a, dBPL/a) and resting period (sBPL/r, dBPL/r); pulse pressure (PP) during 24 hrs (PP/24h), activity (PP/a) and resting period (PP/r); and circadian blood pressure profile and systolic and diastolic blood pressure index during 24 hrs (sBPI/24, dBPI/24), activity (sBPI/a, dBPI/a) and resting period (sBPI/r, dBPI/r). Renal function (serum creatinine level, estimated GFR according to the Schwartz formula), proteinuria, and the use of antihypertensive, renoprotective, and immunosuppressive treatment were analyzed in all children.

* E-mail: pskrzyp@gmail.com

RESULTS: Based on ABPM, hypertension could be diagnosed in 17 patients (36%). Among 30 patients without hypertension in ABPM, six (20%) had elevated (>25%) blood pressure load during 24 hrs, and in another six (20%) elevated blood pressure load was only found during the resting period. Elevated PP was found in 24 (51%) patients. Disturbed circadian blood pressure rhythm was observed in 13 (28%) patients. Proteinuria [mg/kg/24h] correlated positively with sBPI/24h, dBPI/24h, sBPI/a, sBPI/r, dBPI/a, dBPI/r, sBPL/24h, dBPL/24h, sBPL/a, sBPL/r, dBPL/a and dBPL/r. Prednisone doses [mg/kg/24h] correlated positively with sBPI/24h, dBPI/24h, sBPI/a, sBPI/r, dBPI/a, dBPI/r, sBPL/24h, dBPL/24h, sBPL/a, dBPL/a, sBPL/r, and dBPL/r.

CONCLUSIONS: ABPM is a useful method in the evaluation of arterial hypertension in children with various forms of glomerulonephritis. Arterial hypertension, disturbed circadian rhythm of blood pressure and elevated pulse pressure are common findings in children with glomerulonephritis. Higher blood pressure parameters were seen in ABPM in children with more severe proteinuria and in children taking higher prednisone doses.

Introduction

Arterial hypertension is a well-known, the most frequently examined and probably the most important risk factor for progression of all forms of kidney diseases including glomerulopathies [1]. In addition, hypertension is highly prevalent in patients with chronic kidney disease [2]. The prevalence and severity of hypertension correlate with a decrease in glomerular filtration rate (GFR) but these relationships vary depending on the underlying kidney disease [3]. In glomerulopathies, hypertension has been observed to develop already in early stages of the disease, also in patients with preserved GFR. Of particular importance, both chronic kidney disease and chronic inflammatory process (such as in chronic glomerulonephritis) are recognized as conditions associated with significantly accelerated development of atherosclerosis, leading to clinical coronary events occurring already in childhood or during very early adult life [4].

Many hypotheses have been put forward to explain the pathogenesis of hypertension in glomerulopathies. The pathophysiology and the mechanisms leading to the development of high blood pressure in primary glomerular disease are complex and only partially understood. Glomerular injury caused by local inflammation leads to activation of the sympathetic nervous system [5, 6] and the renin–angiotensin-aldosterone system (RAAS), formation of reactive oxygen species, endothelial dysfunction, decreased synthesis of vasodilating substances, sodium retention, and intravascular volume expansion [7, 8, 9].

Increased sympathetic activity is a feature of renally-mediated hypertension and is present in all stages of chronic kidney disease [10]. This phenomenon is probably associated with activation of afferent sympathetic nerves caused by kidney injury [6]. Sympathetic activation leads to both increased cardiac output (stimulation of $beta_1$-adrenergic receptors) and increased peripheral vascular resistance (stimulation of $alpha_1$-adrenergic receptors), thus affecting two main factors determining blood pressure. Studies done in the 1980s demonstrated that in patients with mild deterioration of the renal function, elevation of stroke volume and cardiac output precedes the increase in peripheral resistance [11]. These disturbances are exaggerated by parasympathetic dysfunction developing in the course of the renal disease [6].

Activation of RAAS seems to be a key factor predisposing to further kidney damage and promoting the development of hypertension. RAAS activation is probably responsible for increased secretion of vasoconstricting factors like endothelin-1, with concomitant decrease in synthesis of vasodilating agents like nitric oxide (NO). Angiotensin II leads to high blood pressure not only by increasing smooth muscle tone but also by promoting sodium reabsorption and activation of a number of genes. Angiotensin II activates nuclear factor-kappaB (NF-kappaB), which in turn plays a pivotal role in production and secretion of transforming growth factor beta1 (TGFß-1). TGFß-1 stimulates endothelial cells to synthesize endothelin-1 and inhibits NO production in these cells. The hypothesis of central role of RAAS in the pathogenesis of kidney injury in glomerulopathies is also indirectly supported by renoprotective properties of angiotensin-converting enzyme inhibitors (ACEi) and angiotensin receptor blockers (ARB) [7].

It has also been found that in glomerulopathies more sodium is reabsorbed in cortical common duct cells. This may be at least partially explained by increased activation of sodium-potassium ATPase and endothelial sodium channel (ENaC) in these cells. These two transporters are influenced by many substances (e.g. atrial natriuretic peptide, angiotensin II, NO, prostaglandins, bradykinins), concentrations of which are affected in glomerular kidney diseases. The role of impaired sodium excretion is supported by a very high sodium-sensitivity of hypertension in glomerulopathies [12, 13]. This phenomenon becomes even more evident as renal function deteriorates [14, 15] proportionally to the reduction in number of active nephrons. Impaired sodium excretion is considered to be the most important mechanism responsible for hypertension in chronic kidney disease [9], and increase in blood pressure correlates with expansion of extracellular fluid volume [14].

The prognostic importance of tubulointerstitial changes has been demonstrated in various types of glomerulonephritis. Wehrmann et al. studied 250 cases of focal and segmental glomerulosclerosis and found that the arterial blood pressure correlated with the occurrence of tubulointerstitial changes [16]. Finally, traditional risk factors for hypertension (genetic factors, age, body mass index, diet, insulin resistance) predispose to this complication also in patients with glomerulopathies.

Hypertension is found in 15-80% of adult patients in early stages of chronic glomerulonephritis [3, 17, 18, 19]. The prevalence of arterial hypertension varies depending on the type of glomerular disease, geographical area and the time of the investigation ('new' vs 'old' studies) [7]. Although hypertension may complicate any form of glomerular disease [20], its prevalence depends highly on the type of glomerulopathy. According to Ridao et al., in adults systemic hypertension is most commonly seen in membrano-proliferative glomerulonephritis (GN) (83%), focal and segmental glomerulosclerosis (77%) and in crescentic glomerulonephritis (75%), while it is quite rare in idiopathic nephrotic syndrome (24%) [3]. Arterial hypertension is also present in 20-80% of adult patients with secondary glomerulonephritis with the highest prevalence in Goodpasture's syndrome and diabetic nephropathy. Contreras et al. found that arterial hypertension is one of the most important risk factors associated with poor outcome in patients with lupus nephritis [21]. In addition, Lochynska et al. found that arterial hypertension is significantly more common in adult patients with nephrotic syndrome compared to those without nephrotic range proteinuria [22]. Moreover, the same group showed disturbed circadian rhythm of blood pressure by ambulatory monitoring in 70% of patients with primary GN [23].

IgA nephropathy (IgAN) is the most common glomerulonephritis in adults and it is also a very common condition in pediatric population worldwide [24, 25]. Nephropathy occurs in 20-60% of patients with Schoenlein-Henoch purpura (SHN – Schoenlein-Henoch nephropathy), more commonly in older children [26]. The latter also shares many similarities with IgAN (e.g. IgA deposits in mesangium) and thus these two diseases are frequently evaluated together [27]. Arterial hypertension is found in 19-53% of adult patients with IgA nephropathy at the time of diagnosis. Along with renal function impairment and severe proteinuria, it is the strongest predictor of an unfavorable outcome [28].

Hypertension and proteinuria are the main risk factors for progression of chronic kidney disease in glomerulopathies. Elevated systemic blood pressure transmitted to the glomerular capillary bed increases hyperfiltration and proteinuria, leading to mesangial proliferation, extracellular matrix production, glomerulosclerosis, renal tubule injury, and finally to interstitial fibrosis and irreversible kidney failure.

Twenty-four hour ambulatory blood pressure monitoring (ABPM) is a versatile tool used for analysis of blood pressure parameters in patients with primary and secondary hypertension [29] with very few contraindications (such as severe coagulation disorders, rhythm disturbances, e.g. atrial fibrillation, and, for some brands of equipment, latex allergy) [30]. It has been proven that ABPM is a more precise diagnostic tool that shows better correlation with target organ damage compared to casual blood pressure measurements [31-33]. In patients with chronic renal impairment, regardless of the underlying disease, ABPM is superior to office blood pressure measurements in predicting left ventricular hypertrophy and progression of renal dysfunction [28]. Furthermore, ABPM reveals white coat hypertension, masked hypertension and allows defining diurnal blood pressure variability; it is the only method detecting isolated nocturnal hypertension and abnormal nocturnal dipping, which are very typical features of secondary hypertension [29, 34, 35]. Abnormal ABPM parameters are very common in early stages of glomerulopathies, preceding clinical recognition of hypertension.

Use of ABPM in pediatric patients has grown considerably since early 1990s [29] and currently 63% of pediatric nephrologists reported using this technology in a voluntary survey in 2005 [36]. ABPM is now used successfully in many pediatric centers even in children as young as 2 years of age [36, 37]. Although patients as young as 2 months of age have been studied using 24-hour ABPM, its routine use is usually limited to children aged 5 to 6 years or older [30]. It has been showed that ABPM can be successfully used in pediatric population with sufficient reliability [38] and reproducibility [39-42]. Despite some limitations regarding age-appropriate equipment (e.g. cuff size, which is a critical variable in the accuracy of BP data [30]) and understanding of normal values, ABPM has become a routinely used procedure for the diagnosis of hypertension in children and adolescents. A recent study of 118 pediatric patients (age 3 to 10 years) with chronic kidney disease revealed higher degree of diagnostic specificity and sensitivity compared to both casual and self measurements of blood pressure [43]. It has also been found that children with higher BP values by ABPM are more likely to have increased carotid intima-media thickness [44, 45] and left ventricular hypertrophy [46].

To our knowledge, only very few studies have been performed worldwide to analyze ABPM parameters in children with glomerular kidney disease. Thus, the aim this chapter was to analyze ABPM parameters in such patients. The high prevalence of IgA nephropathy and Schoenlein-Henoch nephropathy together with common blood pressure abnormalities in adult patients with IgAN [47, 48] prompted us to perform specific analyses also in this group of patients.

Patients and Methods

This retrospective study included 47 children with glomerulopathies treated in the Department of Pediatrics and Nephrology at the Medical University of Warsaw. The age range was 4.5 to 18 years (mean age 14.2 ± 3.3 years), and the study population consisted of 26 girls and 21 boys, including 17 patients with IgA nephropathy or Schoenlein-Henoch nephropathy (7 with IgAN, 10 with SHN), 9 with idiopathic nephrotic syndrome, 6 with connective tissue disease or vasculitis (5 with lupus nephritis and 1 with ANCA-positive microscopic vasculitis), 5 with mesangio-proliferative glomerulonephritis, 4 with mesangio-capillary glomerulonephritis, 3 with focal and segmental glomerulosclerosis, 2 with membranous glomerulopathy and 2 with acute post-infectious glomerulonephritis. The diagnosis of glomerular kidney disease was based on clinical symptoms, laboratory findings, and renal biopsy. Mean duration of the disease was 53.2±47.0 months.

Twenty-four hour ABPM was performed in all children. The following standard ABPM parameters were analyzed: systolic, diastolic and mean blood pressure during 24 hours (sBP/24h, dBP/24h, MAP/24h), activity (sBP/a, dBP/a, MAP/a) and resting period (sBP/r, dBP/r, MAP/r); systolic and diastolic blood pressure load during 24 hours (sBPL/24h, dBPL/24h), activity (sBPL/a, dBPL/a) and resting period (sBPL/r, dBPL/r); pulse pressure during 24 hours (PP/24h), activity (PP/a) and resting period (PP/r); and circadian blood pressure profile and systolic and diastolic blood pressure index during 24 hours (sBPI/24, dBPI/24), activity (sBPI/a, dBPI/a) and resting period (sBPI/r, dBPI/r). All blood pressure measurements were compared with BP percentile charts for children and adolescents originally reported by Soergel et al. in 1997 [49], as these are the most widely utilized and the most appropriate (especially for central European children) reference values available [29]. Hypertension was diagnosed when systolic blood pressure and/or diastolic blood pressure during 24 hours was above the 95th percentile for given gender and height. Elevated pulse pressure (PP) was defined as the difference between systolic and diastolic blood pressure exceeding difference between 95th percentile of SBP and 95th percentile of DBP for individual patient. Blood pressure load was calculated as the percentage of readings above a set threshold value (higher than the 95th percentile of blood pressure) for gender and height [50]. Increased systolic or diastolic load was diagnosed when more than 25% of measurements were above the 95th percentile. Disturbed circadian rhythm of blood pressure (i.e., non-dipping) was diagnosed when nighttime systolic or diastolic blood pressure reduction was lower than 10% or blood pressure did not drop at all ([mean daytime BP –

mean nighttime BP]/mean daytime BP x 100). Blood pressure index was calculated by dividing patient's systolic or diastolic blood pressure by 95th percentile of systolic or diastolic blood pressure for individual patient, respectively. 24-hour ABPM was carried out using automatic monitors (SPACELABS 90217 and SCHILLER BR-102) using cuff-oscillometric method. An appropriately sized cuff, as recommended in the Fourth Report on the Diagnosis, Evaluation, and Treatment of High Blood Pressure in Children and Adolescents [51], was placed on the nondominant arm. In all patients, ABPM readings were taken every 15 minutes between 6 a.m. and 10 p.m. and every 30 minutes between 10 p.m. and 6 a.m. The distinction between activity period and resting period was made based on individual patient reports during monitoring (all children were given special diaries to indicate time and duration of activities, as well as child's sleep and wake times). Measurements with less than 80% of valid blood pressure recordings were repeated.

Additionally, renal function (serum creatinine level [mg/dL], estimated GFR according to Schwartz formula [mL/min/1.73 m^2] [52]), daily proteinuria [mg/kg/24 hours], and the use of antihypertensive, renoprotective and immunosuppressive (with glucocorticosteroids) treatment were analyzed in all children. Serum creatinine and proteinuria were assessed using standard laboratory methods. Renoprotective treatment was used in 31 patients (66%), including ACEi in 21 patients (45%), ARB in 1 patient (2%), and double RAAS blockade (ACEi + ARB) in 9 patients (19%). Prednisone was used in 22 patients (47%) in a mean dose of 0.6 mg/kg/24 hours. Ten patients (21%) were treated with immunosuppressive agents: 6 with azathioprine, 3 with cyclosporine A and 1 patient with cyclophosphamide. All patients were on low-sodium diet.

All results are presented as mean values and standard deviation (mean±SD) or as median values (for Mann-Whitney U test). The Mann-Whitney U test was used to examine differences between groups and Spearman-Rank correlation test was used to evaluate correlations between parameters, with $p < 0.05$ considered statistically significant.

Results

Mean GFR in the study group was 140.32±35.74 mL/min/1.73m^2. All patients except for two (children with GFR 63.6 and 61.6 mL/min/1.73m^2, respectively) had normal kidney function. Proteinuria was found in 19 patients (40%). Subnephrotic proteinuria was present in 14 patients (30%). Five patients had nephrotic range proteinuria (11%). Hypertension by ABPM was found in 17 patients (36%). Table 1 shows the prevalence of arterial hypertension and elevated blood pressure load depending on the type of glomerulopathy. Unfortunately, the number of patients with particular forms of glomerulopathy was too small to perform separate statistical analyses (except for combined IgAN and SHN group). We found hypertension in both patients with membranous glomerulopathy, in two third of patients with FSGS and in half of patients with idiopathic nephrotic syndrome, connective tissue and vasculitides, and with mesangio-capillary glomerulonephritis. Elevated blood pressure load during 24 hours was found in 6 patients (13%) and during the resting period only in another 6 patients (13%). Elevated pulse pressure was found in 24 patients (51%), and disturbed circadian blood pressure rhythm in 13 patients (28%).

Table 1. Hypertension prevalence and blood pressure load in patients with different glomerulopathies

Glomerulopathy	AH	Normal BP			Total
		Normal BPL	↑BPL/24h	↑BPL/r	
IgA/Schoenlein-Henoch nephropathy	4 (24%)	9 (52%)	2 (12%)	2 (12%)	17
Idiopathic nephrotic syndrome	4 (50%)	0	2 (25%)	2 (25%)	8
Connective tissue diseases and vasculitides	3 (50%)	3 (50%)	0	0	6
Mesangio-proliferative GN	0	1 (20%)	2 (40%)	2 (40%)	5
Mesangio-capillary GN	2 (50%)	2 (50%)	0	0	4
Focal and segmental glomerulosclerosis	2 (67%)	1 (33%)	0	0	3
Membranous GN	2 (100%)	0	0	0	2
Acute GN	0	2 (100%)	0	0	2
Overall	17 (36%)	18 (38%)	6 (13%)	6 (13%)	47

AH – arterial hypertension
BP – blood pressure
BPL - blood pressure load
r - resting period
GN – glomerulonephritis.

We found positive correlations between prednisone dose [mg/kg/24h] and blood pressure values presented as blood pressure indices and blood pressure load during 24 hours, resting and activity period in patients treated with prednisone. These correlations are presented in Table 2. Additionally, positive correlations between proteinuria and blood pressure parameters presented as blood pressure indices, as well as blood pressure load during 24 hours, resting and activity period were found in patients with proteinuria, as shown in Table 3. We also analyzed the same parameters in a subgroup of patients with IgAN and SHN (overall 17 patients). In these patients, mean GFR was 146.6±25.6 mL/min./1.73m^2. None of these patients had GFR below 90 mL/min./1.73m^2. Proteinuria was found in 7 patients (41%) with IgAN and SHN, subnephrotic proteinuria in 6 patients (35%), and nephrotic range proteinuria in 1 patient (6%). Renoprotection was used in 14 patients (82%), including ACEi in 7 patients (41%), and ACEi + ARB also in 7 patients (41%). Prednisone was used in 8 patients (47%). The mean dose of prednisone was 0.53 mg/kg/24 hours. Five of these patients were treated with immunosuppressive agents, including 4 with azathioprine, and one with cyclophosphamide. Hypertension by ABPM was found in 4 patients (24%). Elevated blood pressure load during 24 hours was found in 2 patients (13%) and in other 2 patients (13%) during the resting period only. Elevated pulse pressure was diagnosed in 9 patients (53%). Disturbed circadian blood pressure rhythm was seen in 3 patients (18%).

Table 2.Correlations between the prednisone dose and ABPM parameters

Parameter	R	p
sBPI/24h	0.64	p<0.005
dBPI/24h	0.59	p<0.05
sBPI/a	0.59	p<0.005
dBPI/a	0.52	p<0.05
sBPI/r	0.54	p<0.01
dBPI/r	0.59	p<0.005
sBPL/24h	0.50	p<0.005
dBPL/24h	0.51	p<0.05
sBPL/a	0.47	p<0.005
dBPL/a	0.47	p<0.05
sBPL/r	0.47	p<0.05
dBPL/r	0.59	p<0.005

sBP - systolic blood pressure
dBP – diastolic blood pressure
I – blood pressure index
L – blood pressure load
a – activity period
r – resting period.

Table 3. Correlations between proteinuria and ABPM parameters

Parameter	R	p
sBPI/24h	0.69	p<0.005
dBPI/24h	0.64	p<0.005
sBPI/a	0.65	p<0.005
dBPI/a	0.58	p<0.01
sBPI/r	0.74	p<0.0005
dBPI/r	0.73	p<0.0005
sBPL/24h	0.65	p<0.005
dBPL/24h	0.63	p<0.005
sBPL/a	0.59	p<0.01
dBPL/a	0.51	p<0.05
sBPL/r	0.73	p<0.0005
dBPL/r	0.68	p<0.005

sBP - systolic blood pressure
dBP – diastolic blood pressure
I – blood pressure index
L – blood pressure load
a – activity period
r – resting period.

Similar positive correlations of ABPM parameters with proteinuria and prednisone were also seen in this subgroup of patients, although they were found only for diastolic blood pressure index (proteinuria: R = 0.46, p = 0.06; prednisone dose: R = 0.59, p<0.05) and diastolic blood pressure load (proteinuria: R = 0.44, p = 0.06; prednisone dose: R = 0.55, p<0.05) during the resting period.

We compared ABPM parameters in groups with or without proteinuria, prednisone treatment and renoprotective treatment using the Mann-Whitney U test. Results of these comparisons are shown in Table 4.

We found no significant differences in ABPM parameters between patients with or without renoprotective treatment in our study.

Table 4. Mean ABPM parameters in patients with or without proteinuria, in patients taking or not taking prednisone, and in patients taking or not taking renoprotective agents (median values)

	Proteinuria vs. no proteinuria	**Prednisone vs. no prednisone**	**Renoprotection vs. no renoprotection**
Number of patients	19 vs. 28	22 vs. 25	31 vs. 16
sBPI/24h	0.947 vs. 0.931 (NS)	0.967 vs. 0.895 (P<0.005)	0.938 vs. 0.906 (NS)
dBPI/24h	0.934 vs. 0.895 (NS)	1.007 vs. 0.868 (P<0.005)	0.918 vs. 0.895 (NS)
sBPI/a	0.925 vs. 0.898 (NS)	0.967 vs. 0.876 (P<0.005)	0.911 vs. 0.892 (NS)
dBPI/a	0.905 vs. 0,833 (NS)	0.952 vs. 0.824 (P<0.05)	0.859 vs. 0.857 (NS)
sBPI/r	0.912 vs. 0.908 (NS)	0.937 vs. 0.857 (P<0.005)	0.892 vs. 0.914 (NS)
dBPI/r	0.985 vs. 0.881 (NS)	0.978 vs. 0.857 (P<0.01)	0.955 vs. 0.866 (NS)
sBPL/24h [%]	18 vs. 14 (NS)	33.5 vs. 9 (P<0.05)	15 vs. 17 (NS)
dBPL/24h [%]	34 vs. 18 (NS)	39 vs. 15 (P<0.01)	20 vs. 18 (NS)
sBLP/a [%]	18 vs. 12 (NS)	27.5 vs. 7.5 (P<0.05)	12 vs. 18 (NS)
dBLP/a [%]	23 vs. 13 (NS)	28 vs. 11 (P<0.05)	15 vs. 17 (NS)
sBPL/r [%]	7 vs. 9 (NS)	11 vs. 3 (P<0.05)	6 vs. 11 (NS)
dBPL/r [%]	41 vs. 15 (NS)	38 vs. 6 (P<0.0005)	23.1 vs. 9 (NS)
Elevated PP [% of patients]	42.1 vs. 57.1 (NS)	54.5 vs. 48 (NS)	51.6 vs. 50 (NS)
sBP dipping [%]	12.6 vs. 11.9 (NS)	11.5 vs. 12.6 (NS)	12.6 vs. 12.0 (NS)
dBP dipping [%]	19.6 vs. 17.9 (NS)	15.9 vs. 19.4 (NS)	17.5 vs. 19.4 (NS)
MAP dipping [%]	18.5 vs. 16.3 (NS)	14.9 vs. 17.8 (NS)	15.9 vs. 19.6 (NS)

MAP - mean arterial pressure
sBP - systolic blood pressure
dBP – diastolic blood pressure
I – blood pressure index
L – blood pressure load
a – activity period
r – resting period.

Discussion

This chapter revealed that arterial hypertension is very common (36%) in children and adolescents with glomerulopathies with normal kidney function. We also found that elevated blood pressure load is a common phenomenon among patients with normal blood pressure by ABPM, revealed in 26% of patients. Additionally, we showed that elevated pulse pressure and disturbed circadian blood pressure profile occur very frequently in these patients (51% and 28%, respectively). Finally, we showed that proteinuria and prednisone dose correlated positively with blood pressure values presented as indices and loads. Of note, in patients with IgAN and SHN these clinical parameters correlated only with diastolic blood pressure during the resting period.

High prevalence of hypertension seen in the study group (36%) is comparable to the prevalence of hypertension in adult patients in early stages of glomerulopathies and is much higher compared to peers without glomerulopathy (1-5%) [51, 53, 54]. Our results also suggest that the type of glomerulonephritis affects the prevalence of hypertension in pediatric population, similarly to what was previously demonstrated in adult patients [3, 8, 9]. Increased blood pressure in these patients can not be explained by decrease in renal function because GFR was reduced in only 2 patients in the study group. We did not evaluate the sympathetic system activity in our patients but there have been many studies (in adult patients) showing increased sympathetic activity in early stages of glomerulopathies [5]. Apart from 36% of our patients with established hypertension, another 26% had elevated blood pressure load during 24 hours or during the resting period. These patients are also at high risk of developing arterial hypertension in the near future. Sorof et al. demonstrated a significantly higher prevalence of left ventricular hypertrophy in children with elevated blood pressure load [55].

Studies performed in the recent years showed higher cardiovascular risk in patients with higher pulse pressure [56]. Elevated pulse pressure is considered to be an independent marker of cardiovascular risk in adult patients with arterial hypertension [57, 58] and chronic kidney disease [59, 60]. Studies performed in adult patients demonstrated a high correlation between pulse pressure and left ventricular hypertrophy [62, 63]. The height of pulse pressure increases as arterial wall compliance diminishes. Elevated pulse pressure is generally associated with arterial stiffness which results in pulsatile blood flow and high systolic-diastolic amplitude [63], thus leading to impaired coronary perfusion [64]. Arterial stiffness is related to high cardiovascular mortality and morbidity and can be caused by atherosclerotic plaques or intramural vascular calcifications. Our study group consisted of children and adolescents with (except for two patients) normal kidney function. In our opinion, the high prevalence of elevated pulse pressure seen in this study can be explained at least partially, as mentioned above, by sympathetic activation, as it mainly increases systolic blood pressure [5]. We believe that similarly to other populations, elevated pulse pressure in children with glomerulopathies may also be a cardiovascular risk factor [65]. Thus, high prevalence of elevated pulse pressure (51%) in our study may suggest high cardiovascular risk in these patients.

Disturbed or even reversed circadian blood pressure profile is a typical feature of secondary hypertension [34, 35]. The presence of this phenomenon should prompt clinicians to perform a thorough search for treatable causes of hypertension [35]. Abnormal night BP pattern is a well-known phenomenon in children with chronic kidney disease, in pre-dialysis stage, during dialysis treatment and after kidney transplantation [2, 66, 67] and is considered to be an early marker of renal function deterioration [30]. Farmer et al. found elevated blood pressure values during the resting period in 55% of adult patients with different types of kidney disease with serum creatinine below 1.25 mg/dL [68]. Other authors showed elevated blood pressure values, especially during the night, in patients with IgAN with normal GFR compared to healthy individuals [48]. On the other hand, it has been proven that adult patients with disturbed 24-hour blood pressure rhythm are at significantly higher risk of developing target organ damage and clinical complications of hypertension (such as myocardial infarction, stroke, and hypertensive nephropathy) compared to patients with similar blood pressure values but with preserved circadian blood pressure rhythm [60-72]. Similarly, children with decreased nocturnal dipping are more likely to show target organ damage, such as left ventricular hypertrophy [73]. Abnormal circadian blood pressure profile is associated with more severe target organ damage also in adult patients with chronic kidney disease managed conservatively [48, 74]. It has not been yet precisely defined how abnormal blood pressure dipping should be defined in children, therefore adult criteria (<10% for both diastolic and systolic blood pressure) were used in this study. The high prevalence of non-dippers seen in the study group may be due to the presence of a secondary cause of hypertension in these patients, but it may also be another indicator of increased cardiovascular risk. In addition, the use of ABPM provides additional information on circadian pharmacological control of blood pressure that may affect the selection and dosage of antihypertensive medications [30]. In our study group, the percentage of dippers and non-dippers was not different in groups receiving renoprotective agents (which also exert an antihypertensive effect), which might mean that these medications did not restore normal circadian blood pressure rhythm in this group of patients. Cisky et al. showed that ACEi are not effective in restoring normal diurnal blood pressure variation, and also demonstrated that the lack of the blood pressure fall during the night accelerates the decrease in renal function in patients with IgAN [47]. Of note, ACEi and ARB show less effective antihyhypertensive action during the resting period, which may be a result of decreased nighttime renin levels [75, 76]. In a LIFE substudy, non-dipping status was more frequent (p=0.01) in a group given losartan-based treatment compared to atenolol-based treatment [77]. In contrast to these studies, German authors in a small study of 14 children with renal hypertension undergoing ABPM monitoring proved that ramipril was effective in lowering 24-hour average blood pressure while also improving nocturnal dipping [78]. In our opinion, other antihypertensive medications apart from ACEi and ARB (like long-acting calcium channel antagonists) should be considered for appropriate blood pressure control in patients with disturbed circadian blood pressure profile. Some studies highlighted the role of small doses of sympatholytic drugs in reducing excessive activity of the sympathetic nervous system [6] which is considered to be a key factor responsible for disturbed circadian blood profile in patients with renal disease.

Correlations between proteinuria and blood pressure values found in our study may be explained by activation of the sympathetic system and the RAAS in these patients. Other authors also found a higher prevalence of hypertension in adult patients with nephrotic syndrome [79]. Rahman et al. evaluated sympathetic activity (by measuring secretion and clearance of noradrenaline) in 6 patients with nephrotic syndrome and normal GFR compared to 6 healthy individuals, demonstrating increased noradrenaline secretion in patients with nephrotic syndrome and comparable plasma renin activity, aldosterone, antidiuretin and atrial natriuretic peptide concentrations in both groups. Rahman et al. concluded that increased sympathetic activity is an early phenomenon in kidney disease with proteinuria that precedes other mechanisms associated with hypertension [80]. The prevalence of hypertension in patients with nephrotic syndrome varies depending on its pathomechanism. In some patients, increased sodium and water reabsorption is a primary mechanism leading to hypervolemia and thus to hypertension. This is often called the "overfill mechanism" and is commonly seen in adult patients with nephrotic proteinuria. In other patients, hypoalbuminemia caused by large urinary protein loss leads to hypovolemia with concomitant sympathetic hyperactivity, the RAAS stimulation and increased aldosterone and antidiuretin secretion. These patients tend to have normal or even low blood pressure values. This so-called "underfill mechanism" is considered to be present in children with idiopathic nephrotic syndrome.

Correlations we found for the prednisone dose may be related to the effect of glucocorticosteroids on blood pressure (e.g. by sensitizing vascular smooth muscle cells to noradrenaline), or to the fact that prednisone was generally used in more severe glomerulopathies. Nevertheless, both these correlations (i.e. with proteinuria and with the prednisone dose) let us conclude that higher blood pressure values by ABPM may be regarded a predictor of a worse clinical course of glomerulopathies. In addition, positive correlations seen only with diastolic blood pressure index and load during the resting period in children and adolescents with IgAN and SHN indicate that these ABPM parameters may be specific prognostic factors of a worse clinical course in this group of patients. Of course, the latter conclusion should be confirmed in a larger group of patients.

To summarize, our finding suggest that glomerular kidney disease is a very strong risk factor for hypertension in children and blood pressure values need to be regularly monitored in these patients. In our opinion, as also supported by our clinical experience, ABPM is a very useful method that allows early diagnosis of hypertension and introduction of antihypertensive treatment in this group of patients.

References

[1] Soergel M; Schaeffer F. Effect of Hypertension on the Progression of Chronic Renal Failure in Children. *AJH* 2002, 15, 53–56.

[2] Mitsnefes M; Kimball TR; Daniels SR. Office and ambulatory blood pressure elevation in children with chronic renal failure. *Pediatr. Nephrol.* 2003, 18, 145-149.

[3] Ridao N; Luno J; de Vinuesa SG. Prevalence of hypertension in renal diseases. *Nephrol. Dial Transplant.* 2001, 16, 70-73.

[4] Kavey RW; Allada V; Daniels SR; Hayman LL; McCrindle BW; Newburger JW; Parekh RS; Steinberger J. Cardiovascular Risk Reduction in High-Risk Pediatric Patients. A Scientific Statement From the American Heart Association Expert Panel on Population and Prevention Science; the Councils on Cardiovascular Disease in the

Young, Epidemiology and Prevention, Nutrition, Physical Activity and Metabolism, High Blood Pressure Research, Cardiovascular Nursing, and the Kidney in Heart Disease; and the Interdisciplinary Working Group on Quality of Care and Outcomes Research. *Circulation.* 2006, 114, 2710-2738.

[5] Ishii M; Ikeda T; Takagi M; Sugimoto T; Atarashi K; Igari T; Uehara Y; Matsuoka H; Hirata Y; Kimura K; Takeda T; Murao S. Elevated plasma catecholamines in hypertensives with primary glomerular diseases. *Hypertension.* 1983, 5, 545-551.

[6] Rump LC; Amman K; Orth S; Ritz E. Sympathetic overactivity in renal disease: a window to understand progression and cardiovascular complications of uremia? *Nephrol. Dial. Transplant.* 2000, 15, 1735-1738.

[7] Kes P; Ljutić D. The role of arterial hypertension in the progression of non-diabetic glomerular diseases. *Nephrol. Dial Transplant..* 2003, 18 [Suppl 5], 28–30.

[8] MacKenzie HS; Taal MW; Luyckx VA; Brenner BM. Adaptation to nephron loss. In: Brenner BM. *The Kidney* Philadelphia: WB Saunders Comp; 2000; 1901-1942.

[9] Naris G; de Jong PE; de Zeeuw D. Renal disease In: Oparil S; Weber MA. *Hypertension* Philadelphia: WB Saunders Comp; 2000; 524-531.

[10] Converse RL; Jacobson TN ; Toto RD; Jost CM; Cosentino F ; Fouad-Tarazi F ; Victor RG. Sympathetic overactivity in patients with chronic renal failure. *N. Eng. J. Med.* 1992, 327, 1912-1918.

[11] Brod J; Bahlmann J; Cachovan M; Pretschner P. Development of hypertension in renal disease. *Clin. Sci.* 1983, 64, 141-152.

[12] Cianciaruso B; Bellizzi V; Minutolo R; Colucci G; Bisesti V; Russo D; Conte G; De Nicola L. Renal adaptation to dietary sodium restriction in moderate renal failure resulting from chronic glomerular disease. *J. Am. Soc. Nephrol.* 1996, 7, 306–313.

[13] Konishi Y; Okada N; Okamura M; Morikawa T; Okumara M; . Sodium sensitivity of blood pressure appearing before hypertension and related to histological damage in immunoglobulin A nephropathy. *Hypertension* 2001, 38, 81–85.

[14] Koomans HA; Roos JC; Boer P; Geyskes GG; Dorhout Mees EJ. Salt sensitivity of blood pressure in chronic renal failure. Evidence for renal control of body fluid distribution in man. *Hypertension* 1982, 4, 190–197.

[15] Kumagai H; Onoyama K; Fujishima M. Effects of salt restriction on blood volume, hemodynamics and humoral factors in patients with chronic glomerulonephritis. *Am. J. Hypertens* 1989, 2, 669–674.

[16] Wehrmann M; Bohle A, Held H; Schumm G; Kendziorra H; Pressler H. Long-term prognosis of focal sclerosing glomerulonephritis. An analysis of 250 cases with particular regard to tubulointerstitial chances. *Clin. Nephrol.* 1990, 33, 115–122.

[17] Martinez-Maldonado M. Role of hypertension in the progression of chronic renal disease. *Nephrol. Dial Transplant.* 2001, 16 [Suppl 1], 63–66.

[18] Malafronte P; Gianna Mastroianni-Kirsztajn G; Betonico GN; Romao JE Jr.; Alves MA; Carvalho MF; Viera Neto OM; Cadaval MA; Bergamo RR; Woronik V; Sens YA; Marrocos MS; Barros RT. Paulista registry of glomerulonephritis: 5-year data report. *Nephrol. Dial Transplant.* 2006, 21, 3098–3105.

[19] Iseki K; Ikemiya Y; Fukiyama K. Blood pressure and risk of end-stage renal disease in a screened cohort. *Kidney Int.* 1996, 49 [Suppl. 55], 69-71.

[20] Anderson Jr. GH; Blakeman N; Streeten DH. The effect of age on prevalence of secondary forms of hypertension in 4.429 consecutively referred patients. *J. Hypertens.* 1994, 12, 609– 612.

[21] Contreras G; Pardo V; Cely C; Borja E; Hurtado A; De La Cuesta C; Iqbal K; Lenz O; Asif A; Nahar N; Leclerq B; Leon C; Schulman I; Ramirez-Seijas F; Paredes A; Cepero A; Khan T; Pachon F; Tozman E; Barreto G; Hoffman D; Almeida Suarez M; Busse JC; Esquenazi M; Esquenazi A; Garcia Mayol L; Garcia Estrada H. Factors associated with poor outcomes in patients with lupus nephritis. *Lupus* 2005, 14, 890—895.

[22] Lochynska K; Oko A; Pawlaczyk K; Krupa D; Simachowicz A; Czekalski S. Incidence of arteria hypertension in early stages of chronic glomerulonephritis. *Nefrol. Dial. Polska.* 2003, 7, 37-40.

[23] Lochynska K; Oko A; Idasiak-Piechocka I; Czekalski S. Circadian rhythm of blood pressure in patients with early phase of primery chronic glomerulonephritis. *Nadcisnienie tetnicze* 2003, 7, 7-14.

[24] D'Amico G. Natural history of idiopathic IgA nephropathy: role of clinical and histological prognostic factors. *Am. J. Kidney Dis.*, 2000, 36, 227–237.

[25] Floege J; Feehally J. IgA nephropathy: recent developments. *J. Am. Soc. Nephrol.,* 2000, 11, 2395–2403.

[26] Hadman JM; Barqawi MA. Henoch-Schoenlein purpura in children. Influence of age on the incidence of nephritis and arthritis. *Saudi Med. J.* 2008, 29, 549-552.

[27] Sanders JT; Wyatt RJ. IgA nephropathy and Henoch-Schoenlein purpura nephritis. *Curr. Opin. Pediatr.* 2008, 20, 163-170.

[28] Nagy J; Kovacs T; Wittmann I. Renal protection in IgA nephropathy requires strict blood pressure control. *Nephrol. Dial Transplant.* 2005, 20, 1533–1539.

[29] Acosta AA; McNiece KL. Ambulatory blood pressure monitoring: a versatile tool for evaluating and managing hypertension in children. *Pediatr. Nephrol.* 2008, 23, 1399-1408.

[30] Urbina E; Alpert B; Flynn J; Hayman L; Harschfield GA; Jacobson M; Mahoney L; McCrindle B; Mietus-Snyder M; Steinberger J; Daniels S. Ambulatory blood pressure monitoring in children and adolescents: recommendations for standard assessment: a scientific statement from the American heart association atherosclerosis, hypertension, and obesity in youth committee of the council on cardiovascular disease in the young and the council for high blood pressure research. *Hypertension* 2008, 52, 433-451.

[31] Devereux RB; Koren MJ; de Simone G; Roman MJ; Laragh JH. Left ventricular mass as a measure of preclinical hypertensive disease. *Am. J. Hypertens* 1992, 5 [suppl], 175-185.

[32] White WB; Schulman P; McCabe EJ; Dey HM. Average daily blood pressure, not office pressure determines cardiac function in patients with hypertension. *JAMA* 1989, 261, 837-877.

[33] Zakopoulos N; Stamatelopoulos S; Toumanidis S; Saridakis N; Trika C; Moulopoulos S. 24h blood pressure profile affects the left ventricle independently of the pressure level. A study in untreated Essentials hypertension diagnosed by office blood pressure Reading. *Am. J. Hypertens* 1997, 10, 168-174.

[34] White WB; Dey HM; Schulman P. Assesment of the daily blood pressure load as a determinant of cardiac function in patients with mild-to-moderate hypertension. *Am. Heart. J.* 1989, 13, 241-244.

[35] Seeman T; Palyzova D; Dusek J; Janda J. Reduced nocturnal blood pressure dip and sustained nighttime hypertension are specific markers of secondary hypertension. *J. Pediatr.* 2005, 147, 366-371.

[36] Woroniecki RP; Flynn JT. How are hypertensive children evaluated and managed? A survey of North American pediatric nephrologists. *Pediatr. Nephrol.* 2005, 20, 791-797.

[37] Varda NM; Gregoric A. Twenty-four-hour ambulatory blood pressure monitoring in infants and toddlers. *Pediatr. Nephrol.* 2005, 20, 798-802.

[38] Wang X; Poole JC; Treiber FA; Harshfield GA; Hanevold CD; Snieder H. Ethnic and gender differences in ambulatory blood pressure trajectories: results from a 15-year longitudinal study in youth and young adults. *Circulation.* 2006, 114, 2780-2787.

[39] Portman RJ; Yetman RJ. Clinical uses of ambulatory blood pressure monitoring. *Pediatr. Nephrol.* 1994, 8, 367-376.

[40] Sorof JM; Portman RJ. Ambulatory blood pressure monitoring in the pediatric patient. *Pediatrics* 2000,136, 578-586.

[41] Lurbe A; Aguilar F; Gomez A; Tacons J; Alvarez V; Redon J. Reproducibility of ambulatory blood pressure monitoring in children. *J. Hypertens.* 1993, 11 [Suppl 5], 288-289.

[42] Stergiou GS; Alamara CV; Salgami EV; Vaindirlis IN; Dacou-Voutetakis C; Mountokalakis TD. Reproducibility of home and ambulatory blood pressure in children and adolescents. *Blood Press Monit.* 2005, 10, 143-147.

[43] Wuehl E; Hadtstein C; Mehls O; Schaefer F. Escape Trial Group. Home, clinic and ambulatory blood pressure monitoring in children with chronic renal failure. *Pediatr. Res.* 2004, 55, 492-497.

[44] Lande MB; Carson NL; Roy J; Meagher CC. Effects of childhood primary hypertension on carotid intima media thickness: a matched controlled study. *Hypertension* 2006, 48, 40-44.

[45] Stabouli S ; Kotsis V; Papamichael C, Constantopoulos A; Zakopoulos N. Adolescent obesity is associated with high ambulatory blood pressure and increased carotid intimal-medial thickness. *J. Pediatr.* 2005, 147, 651-656.

[46] Sorof JM; Alexandrov AV; Cardwell G. Carotid artery intimal-medial thickness and left ventricular hypertrophy in children with elevated blood pressure. *Pediatrics.* 2003, 111, 61-66.

[47] Cisky B; Kovacs T; Wagner L; Vass T; Nagy J. Ambulatory blood pressure monitoring and progression in patients with IgA nephropathy. *Nephrol. Dial Transplant.* 1999, 14, 86-90.

[48] Stefanski A; Schmidt KG; Waldherr R; Ritz E. Early increase in blood pressure and diastolic left ventricular malfunction in patients with glomerulonephritis. *Kidney Int.* 1996, 50, 1321-1326.

[49] Soergel M; Kirschstein M; Busch C, Danne T, Gellermann J, Holl R, Krull F, Reichert H, Reusz GS, Rascher W. Oscillometric twenty-four-hour ambulatory blood pressure

values in healthy children and adolescents: a multicenter trial including 1141 subjects. *J. Pediatr.* 1997, 130, 178-184.

[50] Koshy S; MacArthur C; Luthra S; Gajaria M; Geary D. Ambulatory blood pressure monitoring: mean blood pressure and blood pressure load. *Pediatr. Nephrol.*. 2005, 20, 1484-1486.

[51] Falkner B; Daniels SR; Flynn JT; Gidding S; Green LA; Ingelfinger JR; Lauer RM; Morgenstern BZ; Portman RJ; Prineas RJ; Rocchini AP; Rosner B; Sinaiko AR; Stettler N; Urbina E; Roccella EJ; Hoke T; Hunt CE; Pearson G. National High Blood Pressure Educational Program Working Group on High Blood Pressure in Children and Adolescents. The Fourth Report on the Diagnosis, Evaluation, and Treatment of High Blood Pressure in Children and Adolescents. *Pediatrics* 2004, 114 [Suppl 4th Report], 555-576.

[52] Schwartz GJ; Haycock GB; Edelmann CM Jr; Spitzer A. A simple estimate of glomerular filtration rate in children derived from body length and plasma creatinine. *Pediatrics*. 1976, 58, 259-263.

[53] Hansen ML; Gunn PW; Kaelber DC. Underdiagnosis of hypertension in children and adolescents. *JAMA*. 2007, 298, 874-879.

[54] Lande MB; Kaczorowski JM; Auinger P; Schwartz GJ; Weitzman M. Elevated blood pressure and decreased cognitive function among school-age children and adolescents in the United States. *J. Pediatr.* 2003, 143(6), 720–724.

[55] Sorof JM; Cardwell G; Franco K; Portman RJ. Ambulatory blood pressure and left ventricular mass index in hypertensive children. *Hypertension* 2002, 39, 903-908.

[56] Light P. Current understanding of optimal blood pressure goals in dialysis patients. *Curr. Hypertens. Rep.* 2006, 8, 413-419.

[57] Benetos A; Rudnichi A; Safar M; Guize L. Pulse pressure and cardiovascular mortality in normotensive and hypertensive subjects. *Hypertension* 1998, 32, 560-564.

[58] Haider AW; Larson MG; Franklin SS; Levy D. Systolic blood pressure, diastolic blood pressure and pulse pressure as predictors of risk for congestive heart failure in the Framingham Heart Study. *Ann. Intern. Med.* 2003, 138, 10-16.

[59] Amar J; Vernier J; Rossignol E; Bongard V; Arnaud C; Conte JJ; Salvador M; Chamontin B. Nocturnal blood pressure and 24-hour pulse pressure are potent indicators of mortality in hemodialysis patients. *Kidney Int.* 2000, 57, 2485-2491.

[60] Tozawa M; Iseki K; Iseki C; Takishita S. Pulse pressure and risk of total mortality and cardiovascular events in patients on chronic hemodialysis. *Kidney Int.* 2002, 61, 717-726.

[61] Pannier B; Brunel P; el Aroussy; Lacolley P; Safar ME. Pulse pressure and echocardiographic findings in essential hypertension. *J. Hyperten.* 1989, 7, 127-132.

[62] Viazzi F; Leoncini G; Parodi D; Ravera M; Ratto E; Vettoretti S; Tomolillo C; Sette MD; Bezante GP; Deferrari G; Pontremoli R. Pulse pressure and subclinical cardiovascular damage in primary hypertension. *Nephrol. Dial. Transplant.* 2002, 17, 1779-1785.

[63] Lekakis JP; Zakopoulos NA; Protegorou AD; Papaioannou TG; Kotsis VT; Pitiriga VCh; Tsitsirikos MD; Stamatelopoulos KS; Papamichael CM; Mavrikakis ME. Arterial

stiffness assessed by pulse wave analysis in essential hypertension: relation to 24-h blood pressure profile. *Int. J. Cardiol.* 2005, 102, 391-395.

[64] Fernandez-Fresnedo G; Rodrigo E; de Francisco AL; de Castro SS; Castaneda O; Arias M. Role of pulse pressure on cardiovascular risk in chronic kidney disease patients. *J. Am. Soc. Nephrol.* 2006, 17 [12 Suppl. 3], 246-249.

[65] Leoncini G; Ratto E; Viazzi F; Vaccaro V; Parodi A; Falqui V; Conti N; Tomolillo C; Deferrari G; Pontremoli R. Increased ambulatory arterial stiffness index is associated with target organ damage in primary hypertension. *Hypertension.* 2006, 48, 397-403.

[66] Ozcakar ZB; Yalcinkaya F; Tutar E; Cakar N, Ucar T; Elhan A; Acar B; Yueksel S; Uncu N; Kara N; Atalay S; Ekim M. Hypertension and left ventricular hypertrophy in pediatric peritoneal dialysis patients: ambulatory blood pressure monitoring and ecchocardiographic evaluation. *Nephron Clin. Pract.* 2006, 104, 101-106.

[67] Seeman T; Dusek J; Vondrak K; Simkova E; Kreisinger J; Feber J; Janda J. Ambulatory blood pressure monitoring in children after renal transplantation. *Transplant Proc.* 2004, 36, 1355-1356.

[68] Farmer CK; Goldsmith DJ; Cox J; Dallyn P; Kingswood JC; Sharpstone P. An investigation of the effect of advancing uremia, renal replacement therapy and renal transplantation on blood pressure diurnal variability. *Nephrol. Dial. Transplant.* 1997, 12, 2301-2307.

[69] Palatini P; Penzo M; Racioppa A; Zugno E; Guzzardi G; Anaclerio M; Pessina AC. Clinical relevance of nighttime blood pressure and daytime blood pressure variability. *Arch. Intern. Med.* 1992, 152, 1855-1860.

[70] Verdecchia P; Porcellati C; Schillaci C; Borgioni C; Ciucci A; Battistelli M; Bartoccini C; Porcellati C. Ambulatory blood pressure – an independent predictor of prognosis in essential hypertension. *Hypertension.* 1994, 24, 793-801.

[71] Verdecchia P; Borgioni C; Ciucci A; Gattobigio R; Schillaci G; Sacchi N; Santucci A; Santucci C; Reboldi G; Porcellati C. Prognostic significance of blood pressure variability in essential hypertension. *Blood Pressure Monit.* 1996, 1, 3-11.

[72] White WB. Importance of aggressive blood pressure lowering when it may master most. *Am. J. Cardiol.* 2007, 100, 10-16.

[73] Belsha CW; Wells TG; McNiece KL; Seib PM; Plummer JK; Berry PL. Influence of diurnal blood pressure variations on target organ abnormalities in adolescents with mild essential hypertension. *Am. J. Hypertens.* 1998, 11, 410-417.

[74] Tucker B; Fabbian F; Gilles M; Thuraisingham RC; Raine AE; Baker LR. Left ventricular hypertrophy and ambulatory blood pressure monitoring in chronic renal failure. *Nephrol. Dial. Transplant.* 1997, 12, 724-728.

[75] Schnecko A; Witte K; Lemmer B. Effects of the angiotensin II receptor antagonist losartan on 24-hour blood pressure profiles of primary and secondary hypertension rats. *J. Cardiovasc. Pharmacol.* 1995, 26, 214-221.

[76] Sunaga K; Fujimura A; Shiga T; Ebihara A. Chronopharmacology of enalapril in hypertensive patients. *Eur. J. Pharmacol.* 1995, 48, 441-445.

[77] Bang LE; Wiinberg N; Wachtell K; Larsen J; Olsen MH; Tuxen C; Hildebrandt PR; Ibsen H. Losartan versus atenolol on 24-hour ambulatory blood pressure. A LIFE substudy. *Blood Press.* 2007, 16, 392-397.

[78] Soergel M; Verho W; Wuehl E; Gellermann J; Teichert L; Schaerer K. Effect of ramipril on ambulatory blood pressure and albuminuria in renal hypertension. *Pediatr. Nephrol.* 2000, 15, 113-118.

[79] Kuster S; Mehls O; Seidel C; Ritz E. Blood pressure in minimal change and other types of nephrotic syndrome. *Am. J. Nephrol* 1990, 10 [Suppl. 1], 76-80.

[80] Rahman SN; Abraham WT; Van Putten VJ; Hasbargen JA; Schrier RW. Increased norepinephrine secretion in patients with the nephrotic syndrome and normal glomerular filtration rates: Evidence for primary sympathetic activation. *Am. J. Nephrol.* 1993, 13, 266-270.

In: Hypertension, Heredity and Stroke
Editor: Cristina Moratinos and Bruno Cardenas
ISBN 978-1-60741-496-4

Chapter 5

Surgical Palliative Options for Patients with Hypoplastic Left Heart

***Clifford L. Cua*[1,*]*, *Christopher L. Cua*[2] *and Lillian S. Lai*[3]**
[1]Heart Center, Columbus Children's Hospital;
[2]Section of Thoracic Surgery, Faulkner Hospital;
[3]Section of Cardiology, Children's Hospital of Eastern Ontario.

Abstract

Hypoplastic left heart syndrome (HLHS) was once considered a lethal condition with the two treatment options consisting of hospice care or transplantation; however, with the advent of surgical palliation, first described by Norwood, morbidity and mortality has steadily improved for this patient population. In the current era, three surgical palliations are possible for the initial procedure. These options include: 1) Norwood procedure with pulmonary blood flow supplied via a modified Blalock-Taussig shunt, 2) modification of the Norwood procedure with pulmonary blood flow supplied with a right ventricle to pulmonary artery conduit, or 3) hybrid procedure consisting of bilateral pulmonary artery banding, ductus arteriosus stenting, and balloon atrial septostomy. Each method has certain advantages and disadvantages that make them unique. No method at this time has proven consistently superior and it may be that each procedure has certain advantages over the other depending on the clinical situation and HLHS anatomy. We review the current literature for the three surgical variations with the goal of obtaining a better understanding of the possible surgical options for this complex disease.

* Correspondence concerning this article should be addressed to: Clifford Cua, MD, Heart Center, Nationwide Children's Hospital, 700 Children's Drive, Columbus, OH 43205-2696. Phone: 614-722-2530; Fax: 614-722-2549; clcua@hotmail.com.

Introduction

Hypoplastic left heart syndrome (HLHS) is estimated to occur in approximately 0.162 to 0.267 per 1000 live-births [1]. In the past, it was essentially a lethal congenital heart defect with survival in one natural history study of only 39% within the first week of life [2]. The only two options available for these children were either cardiac transplantation or hospice care. Though transplantation allowed for normal physiology, issues with transplantation included scarcity of pediatric organs, mortality awaiting transplantation, infectious issues, systemic hypertension, chronic immunosuppression, and graft rejection [3-9]. Results from transplantation have steadily improved [10,11], but this option is still impractical for all children with HLHS secondary to organ availability. A surgical palliative procedure was therefore needed and was first described by Norwood [12].

Norwood's first cohort consisted of sixteen patients with nine of the patients undergoing what has become known as the Norwood procedure consisting of anastomosis of the main pulmonary artery to the ascending aorta, aortic arch augmentation, atrial septectomy, and pulmonary blood flow supplied via a central shunt from the newly constructed ascending aorta to the confluence of the pulmonary arteries. This procedure allowed an alternative palliation that theoretically could be performed at any institution; however, there was a 55% (5/9) hospital mortality and a 25% (1/4) late mortality rate [12]. The other seven patients in the original cohort underwent different surgical palliative procedures that were less successful.

One theoretical reason for the high mortality rate in those nine patients included decreased systemic and coronary perfusion due to diastolic run-off of blood flow into the pulmonary arteries through the central shunt. Due to lack of control of pulmonary blood flow with the central shunt, modification of this procedure continued in the ensuring years that eventually resulted in the use of a modified Blalock-Taussig shunt (NW-BT) instead of a central shunt.

Since the NW-BT procedure was first described, initial surgical [13-19], inter-stage [20-22], and second and third stage surgical palliative procedure mortalities [16,19,23-29] have improved. This is likely due to multiple reasons including more experience with dealing with this complex patient population and advances in pre-operative [30], operative [31], and post-operative care [32-36] and technology. Certain risk factors have been implicated that increase morbidity and mortality for the NW-BT procedure and include prematurity, low birthweight, poor ventricular function, diminutive ascending aorta, extracardiac abnormalities, aortic atresia, tricuspid valve insufficiency, coronary artery anatomy abnormalities, cardiopulmonary bypass length, circulatory arrest length, and restrictive atrial septum [15,17,18,37-43]. Again, as more experience has been gained, these risk factors have become less significant [44-46] except for possibly the presence of an intact or highly restrictive atrial septum [47-51]. With all the advances made, initial surgical mortality has decreased significantly in some centers to the high single or mid-teen percentages in the current era [36,45,52]; however, not all centers have been able to duplicate this success with the NW-BT procedure [53-55]. Due to this variability in outcomes and high mortality for certain groups of patients, alternative palliative procedures were thus explored.

One alternative procedure was a modification of the Norwood procedure with pulmonary blood flow being supplied via a right ventricle to pulmonary artery conduit (NW-RVPA) [56-58] which eliminated any diastolic run-off in the systemic circulation. Interestingly, this procedure was also originally described by Norwood in three of his patients, but all three had hospital deaths and thus the procedure was abandoned [12]. The first large cohort to undergo the NW-RVPA procedure in the current era had an initial surgical survival rate of 89% (2/19) compared to a historical NW-BT reference group who had a survival rate of 53% [57]. Since then, other institutions have reported improved surgical survival using the NW-RVPA procedure versus the NW-BT [59-63]; however, other institutions have noted no difference in surgical mortality [45,52,64-66]. The improvement in results by some institutions may be due to the fact that most of these studies used historical NW-BT patients as a comparison group rather than a contemporary one. These studies thus could not account for improvement due to "learning experience" or technical advances. The studies that showed no difference in mortality came from institutions that had relatively low mortality rates with the NW-BT procedure and consequently it would be unlikely that the NW-RVPA procedure would improve mortality significantly.

The main reason given for the improved survival using the NW-RVPA procedure is improved coronary perfusion secondary to higher diastolic blood pressures. All the studies so far comparing hemodynamic variables between the NW-BT and NW-RVPA have documented significantly higher diastolic blood pressures in the NW-RVPA patients [52,60-62,64,67]. The higher diastolic blood pressures are not surprising considering the fact the NW-BT has to and fro flow thru the modified Blalock-Taussig shunt whereas the NW-RVPA has no diastolic run-off because of the neo-aortic valve. Previous studies have shown that one of the reasons for death in these patients may be abnormal coronary anatomy [42,68]; furthermore, children with HLHS have been shown to have abnormal coronary perfusion [69]. One study has documented decreased intensive care and hospital stay and improved enteral feeding [52] but the majority of studies have shown no significant difference in hospital stay [45,60,66]. The improved enteral feeding in the NW-RVPA patients may be another important factor to study considering the high incidence of necrotizing enterocolitis reported for patients undergoing the NW-BT and HLHS patients in general [70,71]. The higher diastolic blood pressures in the NW-RVPA patients would hypothetically improve systemic perfusion [72] and thus the patients would tolerate stressors better in the immediate post-operative period and accordingly have better morbidity and mortality.

The inter-stage time period has also shown significant mortality differences between the two procedures. Multiple studies have shown decreased mortality with the NW-RVPA versus the NW-BT procedure [45,73-78]. Multiple etiologies hypothesized for death during this time period include decreased coronary perfusion, residual arch lesions, shunt/conduit obstruction, arrhythmias, right ventricular failure, and acute intercurrent illness [22,67,68]. Assuming most of the variables would be similar between the two groups, the possible reasons for decreased mortality include improved perfusion and decrease risk for shunt obstruction in the NW-RVPA patients. One study however has shown that inter-stage mortality can be significantly decreased from their original incidence of 15.8% (9/57) to 0% (0/24) in NW-BT patients if a strict home monitoring protocol is instituted [21].

There is conflicting data on the differences in morbidity between these two groups during this time period as well. Some studies have documented no difference in weight at time of the second surgery, age at second stage surgery, need for rehospitalization, or shunt interventions, [45,64,76,79,80] whereas other studies have shown improved weight gain, increased catheterization/surgical interventions, earlier need for second surgery secondary to increase cyanosis, and decreased need for gastrostomy tubes in the NW-RVPA group [45,78,80]. There have also been reports of pseudoaneurysms arising from the site of the RV-PA conduit as well as right ventricular outflow obstruction [66,81-83].

The principal question for the NW-RVPA procedure is what effect an incision has on the right ventricular function long-term. Again, the data from echocardiographic and catheterization studies are contradictory. From a qualitative standpoint, most studies that have compared echocardiographic data between the two procedures have not shown any significant difference in right ventricular function or tricuspid regurgitation [64,78,80,84]. One study did show a trend for worse function and tricuspid regurgitation in the NW-RVPA group long-term, but again this did not reach significance [85]. Another study using strain Doppler echocardiography documented improved longitudinal function in the NW-RVPA group while another study showed similar ventricular efficiency, but decreased contractility in the NW-RVPA patients [83]. Most of the catheterization data obtained before the second stage surgery show increased diastolic blood pressure, decreased systemic saturation, and decreased pulmonary to systemic blood flow ration in the NW-RVPA group [64,79,80,85]. One study showed higher dp/dt ($mmHg/s^2$) in the NW-RVPA group [61]. No study has shown worse right ventricular end diastolic pressure, pulmonary artery pressure, or cardiac index in the NW-RVPA patients [61,78,80]. The McGoon ratio and Nakata index has been noted to be higher in the NW-RVPA patients with more uniform flow to the left and right pulmonary arteries [78,86] though assorted pulmonary artery distortions, especially at the insertion site of the shunt/conduit, have been seen for both procedures [85-88].

The studies comparing stage two results for the two different groups have not shown any significant differences in morbidity or mortality [45,78,80]. Some studies have shown increased incidence of pulmonary artery stenosis in the NW-RVPA group that required pulmonary arterioplasty [59,87], but with modification of the initial NW-RVPA procedure, the incidence of central pulmonary artery stenosis significantly decreased [87]. The length of ventilation, intensive care stay, and hospital stay were equivalent [78,80] and the postoperative hemodynamics for the two groups were essentially the same as well [80]. The three year survival rate for the NW-BT and the NW-RVPA group were similar [45,85]. When stratifying for risk factors, there was no significant difference in type of procedure performed and outcomes; however, there was a trend toward to improved survival in patients with aortic atresia who underwent the NW-RVPA procedure [45].

The only study so far systematically comparing stage three results for the two procedures demonstrated larger pulmonary arteries, more systemic collaterals, higher systemic saturation, and lower systemic pressure and resistance in the NW-RVPA patients. There was no difference in right ventricular end diastolic pressures or qualitative echocardiographic function. There was no difference in length of ventilation, intensive care stay, or hospital stay. There was 100% operative survival [89]. The only other data available comparing post stage three data showed worse echocardiographic function in the NW-RVPA patients [85].

Due to the lack of consistent improvement in morbidity and mortality with the NW-RVPA procedure, the search for an alternative procedure led to the third option for palliation of HLHS patients. Known commonly as the "hybrid" procedure, this procedure consists of bilateral pulmonary artery banding, ductus arteriosus stenting, and balloon atrial septostomy. As early as 1993, stenting of the ductus arteriosus had been described in patients as a bridge to transplantation secondary to the long waiting period [90-92]. This procedure has since evolved into another possibility for HLHS palliation [93-95]. As with the NW-RVPA and NW-BT, advances in technology and experience with this procedure have improved results over time [94,96,97].

The theoretical advantage of this procedure is the ability to avoid a cardiopulmonary bypass run during the neonatal period. Abnormal head size [98], cranial MRI [99,100], cranial ultrasound [101], and fetal cranial blood flow studies [102] have been documented in patients with HLHS before any intervention has been performed and increased cranial ischemic lesions after HLHS surgery have been seen [99,100]. By avoiding bypass during the neonatal period when the cranial vasculature is immature, the hope is that this will improve neurocognitive outcome. This must be weighed against the significantly longer bypass time that is required during the second procedure, which consists of removal of the pulmonary artery bands and ductal stent, anastomosis of the main pulmonary artery to the ascending aorta, aortic arch augmentation, atrial septectomy, and superior vena cavopulmonary connection [94,96,103]. The question of long-term outcome remains unanswered when comparing two bypass runs for the NW pathway during infancy, with one being in the neonatal time period, versus one long bypass run for the hybrid pathway during infancy. The other advantage is that no incision is made into the right ventricle compared to the NW-RVPA procedure and so concerns about long term ventricular function are mitigated. However, the hybrid still has diastolic run-off through the stented ductus similar to the NW-BT, so coronary perfusion could still be theoretically impaired compared to the NW-RVPA.

This procedure was initially performed on high risk patients, as described above, that continued to have significant mortality even in the current era with the NW-RVPA or NW-BT surgery. Mortality or unexpected need for transplantation after hybrid procedure for this high risk group has been reported to be 20% (1 transplantation/5) [104], 21% (3 deaths/14) [103,105], and 60% (9 deaths/15) [106]. When evaluating results from non-high risk patients undergoing this procedure, the mortality rate is significantly lower and has been reported as low as 2.5% (1 death/40) [97] to 18% (2 deaths/11) [107].

The need for postoperative manipulation appears to be less intensive than the NW-RVPA or NW-BT procedure [93,94,108], though one study suggests that this may not necessarily be beneficial for those undergoing the hybrid procedure [108]. This study showed larger fluctuations in systemic and pulmonary vasculature resistance and blood flow, cardiac output, oxygen extraction, and oxygen delivery pre- and post-hybrid compared to the NW-BT. This study also showed no difference in diastolic blood pressures between the two groups. Though the hemodynamics eventually became equal or better than the NW-BT, the authors concluded that some support may be warranted immediately after the hybrid procedure [108]. This institution however routinely placed a 3.5 mm shunt from the innominate artery to the pulmonary artery to prevent loss of flow in the aortic arch and so their results may not be applicable to the hybrid procedure that does not use the "reverse" Blalock-Taussig shunt.

There also continues to be morbidity and mortality during the inter-stage period for this procedure. For the high risk patients, inter-stage mortality has been reported to be 17% (1 death/6) [106], 18% (2 deaths/11) [105], 27% (2 deaths and 1 stage two not pursued secondary to renal dysfunction/11) [103], and 50% (2 deaths/4) [104]. For the non-high risk patients, mortality during this time period ranged from 0% (0/9) [107] to 8% (2 deaths and 1 transplantation/39) [97].

The rate of interventions for this procedure, either surgical or catheter based, range from approximately 30% to 80% [94,97,103,104,106,107,109]. Most of the interventions deal with progressive stenosis of the atrial wall, ductus arteriosus, or isthmus area. Narrowing of the isthmus area, cranially located above the ductus stent, has come to be known as a "retro-coarctation". Interventions described include stenting the atrial septum, placing another stent in the ductus arteriosus, stenting the retro-aortic arch, ballooning the atrial septum, ductus or arch [93,94,96,103,105]. Surgical procedures described include retrieving stents, tightening pulmonary bands, and placing "reverse" Blalock-Taussig shunts [93,94,96,97, 103,105,107,109]. Close surveillance is hence required during this time period to monitor for any of these complications so prompt therapy can be initiated.

Retro-coarctation appears to be the most troublesome issue, especially for patients with aortic atresia since coronary blood flow is entirely dependent on patency of the isthmus area. There is a significant incidence of coarctation previously reported in HLHS patients [110-113] and interventions to relieve this obstruction in the context of the hybrid procedure have met with mixed results [94,97,104,105,109]. If ventricular function is affected by a retro-coarctation and the obstruction is not relieved satisfactorily via catheterization interventions, then the only options available are an early stage two procedure, conversion to a NW, or transplantation. Previous reports have attempted to predict occurrence of coarctation in HLHS patients [114,115] and this should be further investigated because those patients may not be good candidates for the hybrid procedure.

Stage two mortality post hybrid procedure for high risk patients have ranged from 25% (2 deaths/8) [103,105] to 75% (3 deaths/4) [106]. Non-high risk patient mortality ranged from 8% (3 deaths/36) [97] to 11% (1 death/9) [107]. Various interventions consisting of pulmonary arterioplasty as well as extensive arch reconstruction have been reported for this procedure [87,97,103,106]. Timing of this surgery ranged from 3 to 6 months and was institution dependent. The median bypass times reported were 124 [103] to 291 minutes. In general, length of hospital stay did not appear significantly different compared to reported times for the NW-BT or NW-RVPA procedure. Limited data exist for the stage three procedure, but at this time, the available data report no surgical mortality (0/15) [97], (0/4) [103], and (0/11) [96].

Since Norwood first described a surgical palliative treatment for patients with HLHS, significant strides have been made. No comment was even made about current fetal intervention procedures for this patient population. These fetal procedures will no doubt also change future treatment avenues. Multiple options are now available where before there were none. The aspiration continues to be to decrease the morbidity and mortality for this complicated patient population. No option so far as demonstrated superior results. It may be that patients with various anatomical subtypes of HLHS or clinical scenarios would benefit with one procedure over another, but this must be risked assessed. The future objective should be to better delineate this possibility. We look forward to upcoming studies that may answer this question and improve the outcome in this challenging population.

References

[1] Fixler DE, Pastor P, Sigman E, Eifler CW. Ethnicity and socioeconomic status: impact on the diagnosis of congenital heart disease. *J. Am. Coll. Cardiol.* 1993;21:1722-6.

[2] Samanek M. Children with congenital heart disease: probability of natural survival. *Pediatr. Cardiol.* 1992;13:152-8.

[3] Razzouk AJ, Chinnock RE, Gundry SR, et al. Transplantation as a primary treatment for hypoplastic left heart syndrome: intermediate-term results. *Ann. Thorac. Surg.* 1996;62:1-7; discussion 8.

[4] Bove EL. Transplantation after first-stage reconstruction for hypoplastic left heart syndrome. *Ann. Thorac. Surg.* 1991;52:701-4; discussion 704-7.

[5] Zuberbuhler JR, Fricker FJ, Griffith BP. Cardiac transplantation in children. *Cardiol. Clin.* 1989;7:411-8.

[6] Pennington DG, Noedel N, McBride LR, Naunheim KS, Ring WS. Heart transplantation in children: an international survey. Ann. Thorac. Surg. 1991;52:710-5.

[7] Chiavarelli M, Gundry SR, Razzouk AJ, Bailey LL. Cardiac transplantation for infants with hypoplastic left-heart syndrome. *Jama* 1993;270:2944-7.

[8] Jenkins PC, Flanagan MF, Jenkins KJ, et al. Morbidities in patients with hypoplastic left heart syndrome. *Pediatr. Cardiol.* 2004;25:3-10.

[9] Canter C, Naftel D, Caldwell R, et al. Survival and risk factors for death after cardiac transplantation in infants. A multi-institutional study. The Pediatric Heart Transplant Study. *Circulation* 1997;96:227-31.

[10] Bourke KD, Sondheimer HM, Ivy DD, et al. Improved pretransplant management of infants with hypoplastic left heart syndrome enables discharge to home while waiting for transplantation. *Pediatr. Cardiol.* 2003;24:538-43.

[11] Johnston JK, Chinnock RE, Zuppan CW, Razzouk AJ, Gundry SR, Bailey LL. Limitations to survival for infants with hypoplastic left heart syndrome before and after transplant: the Loma Linda experience. *J. Transpl. Coord.* 1997;7:180-4; quiz 185-6.

[12] Norwood WI, Lang P, Casteneda AR, Campbell DN. Experience with operations for hypoplastic left heart syndrome. *J. Thorac. Cardiovasc. Surg.* 1981;82:511-9.

[13] Jonas RA. Intermediate procedures after first-stage Norwood operation facilitate subsequent repair. *Ann. Thorac. Surg.* 1991;52:696-700.

[14] Iannettoni MD, Bove EL, Mosca RS, et al. Improving results with first-stage palliation for hypoplastic left heart syndrome. *J. Thorac. Cardiovasc. Surg.* 1994;107:934-40.

[15] Forbess JM, Cook N, Roth SJ, Serraf A, Mayer JE, Jr., Jonas RA. Ten-year institutional experience with palliative surgery for hypoplastic left heart syndrome. Risk factors related to stage I mortality. *Circulation* 1995;92:II262-6.

[16] Bove EL, Lloyd TR. Staged reconstruction for hypoplastic left heart syndrome. Contemporary results. *Ann. Surg.* 1996;224:387-94; discussion 394-5.

[17] Bando K, Turrentine MW, Sun K, et al. Surgical management of hypoplastic left heart syndrome. *Ann. Thorac. Surg.* 1996;62:70-6; discussion 76-7.

[18] Azakie T, Merklinger SL, McCrindle BW, et al. Evolving strategies and improving outcomes of the modified norwood procedure: a 10-year single-institution experience. *Ann. Thorac. Surg.* 2001;72:1349-53.

[19] Thies WR, Breymann T, Boethig D, Blanz U, Meyer H, Koerfer R. Results of staged reconstruction for hypoplasia of the left heart: an experience of 12 years from one institution. *Cardiol. Young* 2003;13:509-18.

[20] Ghanayem NS, Cava JR, Jaquiss RD, Tweddell JS. Home monitoring of infants after stage one palliation for hypoplastic left heart syndrome. *Semin. Thorac. Cardiovasc. Surg. Pediatr. Card. Surg. Annu.* 2004;7:32-8.

[21] Ghanayem NS, Hoffman GM, Mussatto KA, et al. Home surveillance program prevents interstage mortality after the Norwood procedure. *J. Thorac. Cardiovasc. Surg.* 2003;126:1367-77.

[22] Mahle WT, Spray TL, Gaynor JW, Clark BJ, 3rd. Unexpected death after reconstructive surgery for hypoplastic left heart syndrome. *Ann. Thorac. Surg.* 2001;71:61-5.

[23] Breymann T, Kirchner G, Blanz U, et al. Results after Norwood procedure and subsequent cavopulmonary anastomoses for typical hypoplastic left heart syndrome and similar complex cardiovascular malformations. *Eur. J. Cardiothorac. Surg.* 1999;16:117-24.

[24] Weldner PW, Myers JL, Gleason MM, et al. The Norwood operation and subsequent Fontan operation in infants with complex congenital heart disease. *J. Thorac. Cardiovasc. Surg.* 1995;109:654-62.

[25] Forbess JM, Cook N, Serraf A, Burke RP, Mayer JE, Jr., Jonas RA. An institutional experience with second- and third-stage palliative procedures for hypoplastic left heart syndrome: the impact of the bidirectional cavopulmonary shunt. *J. Am. Coll. Cardiol.* 1997;29:665-70.

[26] Bove EL. Current status of staged reconstruction for hypoplastic left heart syndrome. *Pediatr. Cardiol.* 1998;19:308-15.

[27] Mahle WT, Spray TL, Wernovsky G, Gaynor JW, Clark BJ, 3rd. Survival after reconstructive surgery for hypoplastic left heart syndrome: A 15-year experience from a single institution. *Circulation* 2000;102:III136-41.

[28] Andrews R, Tulloh R, Sharland G, et al. Outcome of staged reconstructive surgery for hypoplastic left heart syndrome following antenatal diagnosis. *Arch. Dis. Child* 2001;85:474-7.

[29] Farrell PE, Jr., Chang AC, Murdison KA, Baffa JM, Norwood WI, Murphy JD. Outcome and assessment after the modified Fontan procedure for hypoplastic left heart syndrome. *Circulation* 1992;85:116-22.

[30] Atz AM, Feinstein JA, Jonas RA, Perry SB, Wessel DL. Preoperative management of pulmonary venous hypertension in hypoplastic left heart syndrome with restrictive atrial septal defect. *Am. J. Cardiol.* 1999;83:1224-8.

[31] Gaynor JW, Kuypers M, van Rossem M, et al. Haemodynamic changes during modified ultrafiltration immediately following the first stage of the Norwood reconstruction. *Cardiol. Young* 2005;15:4-7.

[32] Bradley SM, Simsic JM, Atz AM. Hemodynamic effects of inspired carbon dioxide after the Norwood procedure. *Ann. Thorac. Surg.* 2001;72:2088-93; discussion 2093-4.

[33] Rossi AF, Sommer RJ, Lotvin A, et al. Usefulness of intermittent monitoring of mixed venous oxygen saturation after stage I palliation for hypoplastic left heart syndrome. *Am. J. Cardiol.* 1994;73:1118-23.

[34] Barnea O, Austin EH, Richman B, Santamore WP. Balancing the circulation: theoretic optimization of pulmonary/systemic flow ratio in hypoplastic left heart syndrome. J. *Am. Coll. Cardiol.* 1994;24:1376-81.

[35] Bradley SM, Atz AM, Simsic JM. Redefining the impact of oxygen and hyperventilation after the Norwood procedure. *J. Thorac. Cardiovasc. Surg.* 2004;127:473-80.

[36] Tweddell JS, Ghanayem NS, Mussatto KA, et al. Mixed venous oxygen saturation monitoring after stage 1 palliation for hypoplastic left heart syndrome. *Ann. Thorac. Surg.* 2007;84:1301-10; discussion 1310-1.

[37] Barber G, Helton JG, Aglira BA, et al. The significance of tricuspid regurgitation in hypoplastic left-heart syndrome. *Am. Heart J.* 1988;116:1563-7.

[38] Sauer U, Gittenberger-de Groot AC, Geishauser M, Babic R, Buhlmeyer K. Coronary arteries in the hypoplastic left heart syndrome. Histopathologic and histometrical studies and implications for surgery. *Circulation* 1989;80:I168-76.

[39] Lloyd TR, Marvin WJ, Jr. Age at death in the hypoplastic left heart syndrome: multivariate analysis and importance of the coronary arteries. *Am. Heart J.* 1989;117:1337-43.

[40] Jonas RA, Hansen DD, Cook N, Wessel D. Anatomic subtype and survival after reconstructive operation for hypoplastic left heart syndrome. *J. Thorac. Cardiovasc. Surg.* 1994;107:1121-7; discussion 1127-8.

[41] Kern JH, Hayes CJ, Michler RE, Gersony WM, Quaegebeur JM. Survival and risk factor analysis for the Norwood procedure for hypoplastic left heart syndrome. *Am. J. Cardiol.* 1997;80:170-4.

[42] Vida VL, Bacha EA, Larrazabal A, et al. Surgical outcome for patients with the mitral stenosis-aortic atresia variant of hypoplastic left heart syndrome. *J. Thorac. Cardiovasc.* Surg. 2008;135:339-46.

[43] Nilsson B, Mellander M, Sudow G, Berggren H. Results of staged palliation for hypoplastic left heart syndrome: a complete population-based series. *Acta. Paediatr.* 2006;95:1594-600.

[44] Weinstein S, Gaynor JW, Bridges ND, et al. Early survival of infants weighing 2.5 kilograms or less undergoing first-stage reconstruction for hypoplastic left heart syndrome. *Circulation* 1999;100:II167-70.

[45] Tabbutt S, Dominguez TE, Ravishankar C, et al. Outcomes after the stage I reconstruction comparing the right ventricular to pulmonary artery conduit with the modified Blalock Taussig shunt. *Ann. Thorac. Surg.* 2005;80:1582-90; discussion 1590-1.

[46] Pizarro C, Davis DA, Galantowicz ME, Munro H, Gidding SS, Norwood WI. Stage I palliation for hypoplastic left heart syndrome in low birth weight neonates: can we justify it? *Eur. J. Cardiothorac. Surg.* 2002;21:716-20.

[47] Vlahos AP, Lock JE, McElhinney DB, van der Velde ME. Hypoplastic left heart syndrome with intact or highly restrictive atrial septum: outcome after neonatal transcatheter atrial septostomy. *Circulation* 2004;109:2326-30.

[48] Vida VL, Bacha EA, Larrazabal A, et al. Hypoplastic left heart syndrome with intact or highly restrictive atrial septum: surgical experience from a single center. *Ann. Thorac. Surg.* 2007;84:581-5; discussion 586.

[49] Glatz JA, Tabbutt S, Gaynor JW, et al. Hypoplastic left heart syndrome with atrial level restriction in the era of prenatal diagnosis. *Ann. Thorac. Surg.* 2007;84:1633-8.

[50] Photiadis J, Urban AE, Sinzobahamvya N, et al. Restrictive left atrial outflow adversely affects outcome after the modified Norwood procedure. *Eur. J. Cardiothorac. Surg.* 2005;27:962-7.

[51] Rychik J, Rome JJ, Collins MH, DeCampli WM, Spray TL. The hypoplastic left heart syndrome with intact atrial septum: atrial morphology, pulmonary vascular histopathology and outcome. *J. Am. Coll. Cardiol.* 1999;34:554-60.

[52] Cua CL, Thiagarajan RR, Gauvreau K, et al. Early postoperative outcomes in a series of infants with hypoplastic left heart syndrome undergoing stage I palliation operation with either modified Blalock-Taussig shunt or right ventricle to pulmonary artery conduit. *Pediatr. Crit. Care Med.* 2006;7:238-44.

[53] Jacobs ML, Blackstone EH, Bailey LL. Intermediate survival in neonates with aortic atresia: a multi-institutional study. The Congenital Heart Surgeons Society. *J. Thorac. Cardiovasc. Surg.* 1998;116:417-31.

[54] Gutgesell HP, Gibson J. Management of hypoplastic left heart syndrome in the 1990s. *Am. J. Cardiol.* 2002;89:842-6.

[55] Lofland GK, McCrindle BW, Williams WG, et al. Critical aortic stenosis in the neonate: a multi-institutional study of management, outcomes, and risk factors. Congenital Heart Surgeons Society. *J. Thorac. Cardiovasc. Surg.* 2001;121:10-27.

[56] Kishimoto H, Kawahira Y, Kawata H, Miura T, Iwai S, Mori T. The modified Norwood palliation on a beating heart. *J. Thorac. Cardiovasc. Surg.* 1999;118:1130-2.

[57] Sano S, Ishino K, Kawada M, et al. Right ventricle-pulmonary artery shunt in first-stage palliation of hypoplastic left heart syndrome. *J. Thorac. Cardiovasc. Surg.* 2003;126:504-9; discussion 509-10.

[58] Imoto Y, Kado H, Shiokawa Y, Fukae K, Yasui H. Norwood procedure without circulatory arrest. *Ann. Thorac. Surg.* 1999;68:559-61.

[59] Griselli M, McGuirk SP, Stumper O, et al. Influence of surgical strategies on outcome after the Norwood procedure. *J. Thorac. Cardiovasc. Surg.* 2006;131:418-26.

[60] Mair R, Tulzer G, Sames E, et al. Right ventricular to pulmonary artery conduit instead of modified Blalock-Taussig shunt improves postoperative hemodynamics in newborns after the Norwood operation. *J. Thorac. Cardiovasc. Surg.* 2003;126:1378-84.

[61] Malec E, Januszewska K, Kolcz J, Mroczek T. Right ventricle-to-pulmonary artery shunt versus modified Blalock-Taussig shunt in the Norwood procedure for hypoplastic

left heart syndrome - influence on early and late haemodynamic status. *Eur. J. Cardiothorac. Surg.* 2003;23:728-33; discussion 733-4.

[62] Pizarro C, Malec E, Maher KO, et al. Right ventricle to pulmonary artery conduit improves outcome after stage I Norwood for hypoplastic left heart syndrome. *Circulation* 2003;108 Suppl 1:II155-60.

[63] Tibballs J, Kawahira Y, Carter BG, Donath S, Brizard C, Wilkinson J. Outcomes of surgical treatment of infants with hypoplastic left heart syndrome: an institutional experience 1983-2004. *J. Paediatr. Child Health* 2007;43:746-51.

[64] Azakie A, Martinez D, Sapru A, Fineman J, Teitel D, Karl TR. Impact of right ventricle to pulmonary artery conduit on outcome of the modified Norwood procedure. *Ann. Thorac. Surg.* 2004;77:1727-33.

[65] Bradley SM, Simsic JM, McQuinn TC, Habib DM, Shirali GS, Atz AM. Hemodynamic status after the Norwood procedure: a comparison of right ventricle-to-pulmonary artery connection versus modified Blalock-Taussig shunt. *Ann. Thorac. Surg.* 2004;78:933-41; discussion 933-41.

[66] Mahle WT, Cuadrado AR, Tam VK. Early experience with a modified Norwood procedure using right ventricle to pulmonary artery conduit. *Ann. Thorac. Surg.* 2003;76:1084-8; discussion 1089.

[67] Ghanayem NS, Jaquiss RD, Cava JR, et al. Right ventricle-to-pulmonary artery conduit versus Blalock-Taussig shunt: a hemodynamic comparison. *Ann. Thorac. Surg.* 2006;82:1603-9; discussion 1609-10.

[68] Bartram U, Grunenfelder J, Van Praagh R. Causes of death after the modified Norwood procedure: a study of 122 postmortem cases. *Ann. Thorac. Surg.* 1997;64:1795-802.

[69] Donnelly JP, Raffel DM, Shulkin BL, et al. Resting coronary flow and coronary flow reserve in human infants after repair or palliation of congenital heart defects as measured by positron emission tomography. *J. Thorac. Cardiovasc. Surg.* 1998;115:103-10.

[70] Jeffries HE, Wells WJ, Starnes VA, Wetzel RC, Moromisato DY. Gastrointestinal morbidity after Norwood palliation for hypoplastic left heart syndrome. *Ann. Thorac. Surg.* 2006;81:982-7.

[71] McElhinney DB, Hedrick HL, Bush DM, et al. Necrotizing enterocolitis in neonates with congenital heart disease: risk factors and outcomes. *Pediatrics* 2000;106:1080-7.

[72] Harrison AM, Davis S, Reid JR, et al. Neonates with hypoplastic left heart syndrome have ultrasound evidence of abnormal superior mesenteric artery perfusion before and after modified Norwood procedure. *Pediatr. Crit. Care Med.* 2005;6:445-7.

[73] Cua CL, Thiagarajan RR, Taeed R, et al. Improved interstage mortality with the modified Norwood procedure: a meta-analysis. *Ann. Thorac. Surg.* 2005;80:44-9.

[74] da Silva JP, da Fonseca L, Baumgratz JF, et al. Hypoplastic left heart syndrome: the report of a surgical strategy and comparative results of Norwood x Norwood-Sano approach. *Rev Bras Cir Cardiovasc* 2007;22:160-8.

[75] Pigula FA, Vida V, Del Nido P, Bacha E. Contemporary results and current strategies in the management of hypoplastic left heart syndrome. *Semin. Thorac. Cardiovasc. Surg.* 2007;19:238-44.

[76] Pizarro C, Mroczek T, Malec E, Norwood WI. Right ventricle to pulmonary artery conduit reduces interim mortality after stage 1 Norwood for hypoplastic left heart syndrome. *Ann. Thorac. Surg.* 2004;78:1959-63; discussion 1963-4.

[77] Silva JP, Fonseca L, Baumgratz JF, et al. Hypoplastic left heart syndrome: the influence of surgical strategy on outcomes. *Arq. Bras. Cardiol.* 2007;88:354-60.

[78] Graham EM, Atz AM, Bradley SM, et al. Does a ventriculotomy have deleterious effects following palliation in the Norwood procedure using a shunt placed from the right ventricle to the pulmonary arteries? *Cardiol Young* 2007;17:145-50.

[79] Malec E, Januszewska K, Kolz J, Pajak J. Factors influencing early outcome of Norwood procedure for hypoplastic left heart syndrome. *Eur. J. Cardiothorac. Surg.* 2000;18:202-6.

[80] Lai L, Laussen PC, Cua CL, et al. Outcomes after bidirectional Glenn operation: Blalock-Taussig shunt versus right ventricle-to-pulmonary artery conduit. *Ann. Thorac. Surg.* 2007;83:1768-73.

[81] Cua CL, Sanghavi D, Voss S, et al. Right ventricular pseudoaneurysm after modified Norwood procedure. *Ann. Thorac. Surg.* 2004;78:e72-3.

[82] Sano S, Ishino K, Kado H, et al. Outcome of right ventricle-to-pulmonary artery shunt in first-stage palliation of hypoplastic left heart syndrome: a multi-institutional study. *Ann. Thorac. Surg.* 2004;78:1951-7; discussion 1957-8.

[83] Tanoue Y, Kado H, Shiokawa Y, Fusazaki N, Ishikawa S. Midterm ventricular performance after Norwood procedure with right ventricular-pulmonary artery conduit. *Ann. Thorac. Surg.* 2004;78:1965-71; discussion 1971.

[84] Frommelt PC, Sheridan DC, Mussatto KA, et al. Effect of shunt type on echocardiographic indices after initial palliations for hypoplastic left heart syndrome: Blalock-Taussig shunt versus right ventricle-pulmonary artery conduit. J. Am. Soc. Echocardiogr 2007;20:1364-73.

[85] Ballweg JA, Dominguez TE, Ravishankar C, et al. A contemporary comparison of the effect of shunt type in hypoplastic left heart syndrome on the hemodynamics and outcome at stage 2 reconstruction. *J. Thorac. Cardiovasc. Surg.* 2007;134:297-303.

[86] Rumball EM, McGuirk SP, Stumper O, et al. The RV-PA conduit stimulates better growth of the pulmonary arteries in hypoplastic left heart syndrome. *Eur. J. Cardiothorac. Surg.* 2005;27:801-6.

[87] Nakano T, Fukae K, Sonoda H, et al. Follow-up study of pulmonary artery configuration in hypoplastic left heart syndrome. Gen. Thorac. Cardiovasc. Surg. 2008;56:54-62.

[88] Griselli M, McGuirk SP, Ofoe V, et al. Fate of pulmonary arteries following Norwood Procedure. Eur. J. Cardiothorac. Surg. 2006;30:930-5.

[89] Januszewska K, Stebel A, Malec E. Consequences of right ventricle-to-pulmonary artery shunt at the first stage for the Fontan operation. Ann. Thorac. Surg. 2007;84:1611-7.

[90] Ruiz CE, Gamra H, Zhang HP, Garcia EJ, Boucek MM. Brief report: stenting of the ductus arteriosus as a bridge to cardiac transplantation in infants with the hypoplastic left-heart syndrome. *N. Engl. J. Med.* 1993;328:1605-8.

[91] Boucek MM, Mashburn C, Chan KC. Catheter-based interventional palliation for hypoplastic left heart syndrome. *Semin. Thorac. Cardiovasc. Surg. Pediatr. Card. Surg. Annu.* 2005:72-7.

[92] Slack MC, Kirby WC, Towbin JA, et al. Stenting of the ductus arteriosus in hypoplastic left heart syndrome as an ambulatory bridge to cardiac transplantation. *Am. J. Cardiol.* 1994;74:636-7.

[93] Akintuerk H, Michel-Behnke I, Valeske K, et al. Stenting of the arterial duct and banding of the pulmonary arteries: basis for combined Norwood stage I and II repair in hypoplastic left heart. *Circulation* 2002;105:1099-103.

[94] Galantowicz M, Cheatham JP. Lessons learned from the development of a new hybrid strategy for the management of hypoplastic left heart syndrome. *Pediatr. Cardiol.* 2005;26:190-9.

[95] Michel-Behnke I, Akintuerk H, Marquardt I, et al. Stenting of the ductus arteriosus and banding of the pulmonary arteries: basis for various surgical strategies in newborns with multiple left heart obstructive lesions. *Heart* 2003;89:645-50.

[96] Akinturk H, Michel-Behnke I, Valeske K, et al. Hybrid transcatheter-surgical palliation: basis for univentricular or biventricular repair: the Giessen experience. *Pediatr. Cardiol.* 2007;28:79-87.

[97] Galantowicz M, Cheatham JP, Phillips A, et al. Hybrid approach for hypoplastic left heart syndrome: intermediate results after the learning curve. *Ann. Thorac. Surg.* 2008;85:2063-71.

[98] Manzar S, Nair AK, Pai MG, Al-Khusaiby SM. Head size at birth in neonates with transposition of great arteries and hypoplastic left heart syndrome. *Saudi Med. J.* 2005;26:453-6.

[99] Dent CL, Spaeth JP, Jones BV, et al. Brain magnetic resonance imaging abnormalities after the Norwood procedure using regional cerebral perfusion. *J. Thorac. Cardiovasc. Surg.* 2006;131:190-7.

[100] Dent CL, Spaeth JP, Jones BV, et al. Brain magnetic resonance imaging abnormalities after the Norwood procedure using regional cerebral perfusion. *J. Thorac. Cardiovasc. Surg.* 2005;130:1523-30.

[101] Te Pas AB, van Wezel-Meijler G, Bokenkamp-Gramann R, Walther FJ. Preoperative cranial ultrasound findings in infants with major congenital heart disease. *Acta. Paediatr.* 2005;94:1597-603.

[102] Kaltman JR, Di H, Tian Z, Rychik J. Impact of congenital heart disease on cerebrovascular blood flow dynamics in the fetus. *Ultrasound. Obstet. Gynecol.* 2005;25:32-6.

[103] Pizarro C, Murdison KA, Derby CD, Radtke W. Stage II reconstruction after hybrid palliation for high-risk patients with a single ventricle. *Ann. Thorac. Surg.* 2008;85:1382-8.

[104] Lim DS, Peeler BB, Matherne GP, Kron IL, Gutgesell HP. Risk-stratified approach to hybrid transcatheter-surgical palliation of hypoplastic left heart syndrome. *Pediatr. Cardiol.* 2006;27:91-5.

[105] Bacha EA, Daves S, Hardin J, et al. Single-ventricle palliation for high-risk neonates: the emergence of an alternative hybrid stage I strategy. *J. Thorac. Cardiovasc. Surg.* 2006;131:163-171 e2.

[106] Pilla CB, Pedra CA, Nogueira AJ, et al. Hybrid Management for Hypoplastic Left Heart Syndrome : An Experience from Brazil. *Pediatr. Cardiol.* 2007.

[107] Caldarone CA, Benson L, Holtby H, Li J, Redington AN, Van Arsdell GS. Initial experience with hybrid palliation for neonates with single-ventricle physiology. *Ann. Thorac. Surg.* 2007;84:1294-300.

[108] Li J, Zhang G, Benson L, et al. Comparison of the profiles of postoperative systemic hemodynamics and oxygen transport in neonates after the hybrid or the Norwood procedure: a pilot study. *Circulation* 2007;116:I179-87.

[109] Caldarone CA, Benson LN, Holtby H, Van Arsdell GS. Main pulmonary artery to innominate artery shunt during hybrid palliation of hypoplastic left heart syndrome. *J. Thorac. Cardiovasc. Surg.* 2005;130:e1-2.

[110] Hawkins JA, Doty DB. Aortic atresia: morphologic characteristics affecting survival and operative palliation. *J. Thorac. Cardiovasc. Surg.* 1984;88:620-6.

[111] Jonas RA, Lang P, Hansen D, Hickey P, Castaneda AR. First-stage palliation of hypoplastic left heart syndrome. The importance of coarctation and shunt size. *J. Thorac. Cardiovasc. Surg.* 1986;92:6-13.

[112] Zellers TM. Balloon angioplasty for recurrent coarctation of the aorta in patients following staged palliation for hypoplastic left heart syndrome. *Am. J. Cardiol.* 1999;84:231-3, A9.

[113] Zeltser I, Menteer J, Gaynor JW, et al. Impact of re-coarctation following the Norwood operation on survival in the balloon angioplasty era. *J. Am. Coll. Cardiol.* 2005;45:1844-8.

[114] Boucek MM, Mashburn C, Kunz E, Chan KC. Ductal anatomy: a determinant of successful stenting in hypoplastic left heart syndrome. *Pediatr. Cardiol.* 2005;26:200-5.

[115] Lemler MS, Zellers TM, Harris KA, Ramaciotti C. Coarctation index: identification of recurrent coarctation in infants with hypoplastic left heart syndrome after the Norwood procedure. *Am. J. Cardiol.* 2000;86:697-9, A9.

In: Hypertension, Heredity and Stroke
Editor: Cristina Moratinos and Bruno Cardenas

ISBN 978-1-60741-496-4

Chapter 6

Influence of Heart Rate on Development of Stroke among Patients at Risk for Cerebrovascular Disease

***Basil N. Okeahialam**[*1] **and Ayuba I. Zoakah**[2]*
[1]Department of Medicine
[2]Department of Community Health
Jos University Teaching Hospital, Jos, Nigeria

Abstract

Background: The importance of heart rate as a prognostic factor and potential therapeutic target, despite suggestive evidence has not yet been generally accepted. Whereas drugs that reduce heart rate improve outcome in ischaemic heart disease and congestive cardiac failure, such is said not to be the experience with stroke. It has been reported that uncomplicated hypertension treated with beta blockers is associated with an increase in stroke especially in the elderly. While it is known how raised heart rate adversely affects ischaemic heart disease and congestive cardiac failure, it has not been clearly shown how low heart rate increases tendency to stroke. This report is on studies which suggest that lower heart rate is related to the occurrence of stroke.

Methods: Two cohorts of stroke patients had their heart rates determined clinically. Drugs and diseases likely to affect heart rate served as exclusion criteria. Finally only those in sinus rhythm were enrolled. They were compared with sex and age ($\pm$ 5 years) matched controls on who the same criteria applied along three lines: mean values, proportions along above and below average heart rate lines; as well as in six different heart rate groups. Pair- matched analysis of data was also done.

Results: In the first cohort, the mean heart rate of 77.5 $\pm$ 13.3 per minute was significantly lower than the mean of 90.3 $\pm$ 13.6 per minute among the controls ($t = 3.17$. $p < 0.01$). Along the lines of above and below average, the proportion of stroke patients whose heart rates was below average was significantly higher than the controls (chi

[*] E mail: basokeam@yahoo.com, Phone: 234 0803 7211 698

square with Yates correction = 4.17. $p < 0.05$). When grouped into six, the proportions of the cases was significantly higher than the controls in classes < 60/minute ($t = 2.06$. $p < 0.05$) and 61 – 70/minute ($t = 2.14$. $p < 0.05$). For the class >100/minute, the cases were significantly fewer than the controls ($t = 2.26$. $p < 0.05$).

In the second cohort, the mean heart rate of 78.4 ± 10.4 per minute among cases was lower than, but not significantly from 82.3 ± 8.4 per minute recorded for the controls. However when grouped above or below average, the proportion of stroke patients below average was significantly higher than controls (chi square with Yates correction = 9.08. $p < 0.01$). Along the six group lines, significant difference emerged only in the 61 – 70/minute range, with cases more than controls ($t = 4.38$. $p < 0.0001$).

When pair-matched analysis was done using McNemars's test, the association between stroke cases and low heart rate was highly significant ($p < 0.001$)

Discussion: The lower the heart rate, the more sluggish the circulation. This makes for thrombus formation especially as the arterial tree may have been narrowed from atherosclerotic plaques caused by predisposing diseases. Consequently the chances of ischaemic stroke from thrombo-embolism would be raised especially during periods of inactivity.

Keywords: Heart rate, Stroke, Thrombo-embolism, Ischaemia.

Introduction

Various factors are known to predispose individuals to stroke. While some are major, others are relatively minor. Irrespective of what category a risk factor belongs to, outright removal or manipulative intervention would have a salutary effect on the outcome. This echoes the opinion of Schoenberg [1] that there is greater benefit in dealing with precussors of stroke rather than delaying treatment until after the event. The rising incidence of stroke over the years [2] calls for concern. Completed stroke remains a major cause of morbidity and mortality [3] and represents a considerable burden of work for various members of the health team. The importance of heart rate as a prognostic factor and potential therapeutic target despite suggestive evidence has not yet been accepted generally [4]. Whereas drugs that reduce heart rate like beta blockers improve outcome in ischaemic heart disease and congestive cardiac failure, such is said not to be the experience with stroke [5]. Further more, while it is known how raised heart rate adversely affects ischaemic heart disease and congestive cardiac failure, it has not yet been shown how and if low heart rate increases tendency to stroke.

Cases have been encountered in practice where cerebrovascular disease patients have low heart rate and no major risk factors (Okeahialam BN – Unpublished clinical observations). A few studies however have reported some form of association between bradycardia or low heart rate with stroke [6,7,8], without offering clear explanation. This pilot study was therefore designed to determine if heart rate was associated with development of stroke in patients at risk for cerebrovascular disease; and suggest probable mechanisms.

Patients and Methods

Over a twenty four month period, all patients consecutively admitted with a clinical diagnosis of stroke on the medical service of Jos University Teaching Hospital were examined by one of the authors (BNO). Those in congestive cardiac failure were excluded as were those on either digitalis or beta blocker therapy. This was to remove disease or drug related effect on heart rate. This constituted group A. Any major risk factor for cerebrovascular disease was noted and included hypertension, diabetes mellitus, obesity, and chronic alcohol ingestion. The radial pulse and heart rate by auscultation were each counted for one minute to ensure that there was no significant pulse deficit. Thereafter the pulse rate was used for assessment. A twelve lead resting electrocardiogram was obtained for all patients, and those not in sinus rhythm were excluded. The pulse rate was counted a second time between 10 pm and 2 am while the patients were sleeping. The pulse rate recorded by the admitting doctor was obtained from the case notes, and the mean of the three values was considered representative. This was the value used for analysis as representing heart rate. Admission and hence examination after the cerebrovascular accident varied from hours in a few cases to days and weeks in most and months in another few. To serve as controls, patients on admission in the same wards over the same period, who had diagnosis and treatments unlikely to affect heart rate were assessed in the same way. The time interval between assessment of cases and controls was within five minutes in all instances. Controls were matched for sex and age (± 5 years); and as much as possible for background diseases.

A second group was made up of consecutive post-stroke patients attending the medical out-patient clinics for follow up. They were also examined solely by one of the authors (BNO). Exclusion criteria were background congestive cardiac failure and use of digitalis and beta blockers as for group A. Those meeting the inclusion criteria were enrolled and had their pulse rates counted for one minute provided there was no significant deficit between it and the heart rate counted by auscultation over the praecordium. This was to ensure that patients were in sinus rhythm. The pulse rate documented by the reviewing doctor on the previous visit was extracted from the records. The mean of these two readings was considered representative of heart rate for the patient and used for analysis. This cohort constituted group B. Patients attending the same clinics on same days for conditions other than stroke, and who had no disease or drug therapy that could affect heart rate served as controls. They were matched for sex, age (±5 years) and underlying disease. Their pulse rates were also counted for one minute. As with the main group, the previous clinic visit pulse rates were extracted from the records; and the mean of the two calculated for the patient and used for analysis. Informed consent was given in all cases by patients themselves or by immediate relations in cases of coma or expressive dysphasia.

In our environment we had found (Okeahialam and Anjorin – Unpublished) that the mean pulse rate per minute of a randomly selected sample of the normal population was 80.9 ±0.9 (SE) and for a group of hypertensives 81.5 ±1.4 (SE). However as the average heart at rest is said to beat at 70/minute [9], all patients and controls alike were with 70 as cut off grouped into above and below average. Again, the number of cases and controls for groups A and B were disposed into six pulse rate class ranges. Data were then analysed by one of the authors (AIZ) for statistical significance using chi square, McNemar's and student t- tests where applicable. P value was set at <0.05 for statistical significance.

Results

Fifty two patients satisfied the criteria for group A. Thirty six were males and 16 females, a male to female ratio of 2.25:1. Their ages ranged from 21 to 98 years with a mean of 54.3 years. Only 29 satisfactory controls were studied, 17 males and 12 females giving a male to female ratio of 1.4: 1. Their ages ranged from 30 to 79 years with a mean of 51.7 years. For group B, 66 patients satisfying the inclusion criteria were studied. Fourty five were males and 21 females giving a male to female ratio of 2.14:1. Their ages ranged from 18 to 82 years with a mean of 52.8 years. Fourty eight satisfactory controls were studied, 30 male and 18 females giving a male to female ratio of 1.6: 1. Their ages ranged from 23 to 85 with a mean of 49.7 years.

The mean heart rate of the stroke in-patients in group A was 77.5 $\pm$ 13.3 (SD) while for their controls it was 90.3 $\pm$ 13.6 (SD). The difference was statistically significant at $p< 0.01$ ($t = 3.97$); with the cases lower than the controls. For group B, the out-patient group, the mean heart rate of the stroke cases was 78.7 $\pm$ 10.4 (SD). In contrast, their control group had a mean heart rate of 82.4 $\pm$ 8.7 (SD). Even though the mean heart rate of the stroke cases tended to be lower than that of the controls, the difference did not attain statistical significance.

In group A, 15 of the stroke patients had heart rates below average; while 37 were above average. For their controls, 2 had heart rates below average; while 27 were above average. The difference in proportions was statistically significant, with more stroke cases than controls having heart rates below average. The chi-square value with Yate's correction was 4.17. $p<0.05$. Odds Ratio 5.5. (See Table 1).

In group B, 16 of the stroke patients had heart rates below average and 50 had heart rates above average. Among their controls, only 1 patient had a heart rate below average; while the remaining 47 had heart rates above average.

Table 1. 2 X 2 CONTINGENCY TABLE FOR GROUP A

	Below Average Heart Rate	Above Average Heart Rate	Total
Stroke Cases	15 (10.4)	37 (41)	52
No Stroke Contr.	2 (6.0)	27 (22.9)	29
Total	17	64	81

Chi- squared value (With Yate's correction) = 4.17. df 1 p = 0.04 (< 0.05). OR 5.5
Values outside parentheses are observed and those within parentheses are calculated expected values
df – degree of freedom
OR – Odds ratio.

Table 2. 2 X 2 CONTINGENCY TABLE FOR GROUP B

	Below Average Heart Rate	Above Average Heart Rate	Total
Stroke Cases	16 (9.8)	50 (56.1)	66
No Stroke Contr.	1 (7.1)	47 (40.8)	48
Total	17	97	114

Chi-squared value (with Yate's correction) = 9.08. df 1 p = 0.003 (<0.01) OR = 15

Values outside parentheses are observed while values within parentheses are calculated expected values.

df - degree of freedom

OR – Odds ratio.

The difference in proportions was again statistically significant with more stroke cases than controls having heart rates below average. The chi-square value with Yate's correction was 9.08. p<0.01. Odds Ratio 15. (See Table 2).

Disposing cases from both groups into 6 heart rate class ranges, more of the stroke cases compared with controls were in the lower ranges with varying levels of statistical significance. (See Table 3). When pair matched analysis was done using McNemar's test, the association between stroke (cases) and below average heart rate was highly significant. (See Table 4).

Table 3. COMPARISON OF CASES AND CONTROLS BY HEART/PULSE RATE RANGES

Range of HR	1	2	3	4	5	6
A Cases (n = 52)	4	11	14	14	6	3
Controls (n = 29)	0	2	4	9	7	7
B Cases (n = 66)	3	13	24	19	6	1
Controls (n = 48)	0	1	24	16	5	2

Key: Range 1: ≤ 60/min. Range 2: 61 – 70/min. Range 3: 71 – 80/min.

Range 4: 81 – 90/min. Range 5: 91 – 100/min. Range 6: > 100/min

For group A: Difference in proportions between cases and controls attained statistical significance for Range 1 (≤ 60/min) – t = 2.058. df 79. p< 0.05.

Range 2 (61 – 70/min) – t = 2.142. df 79. p< 0.05

Range 6 (> 100/min) – t = 2.261. df 79. p< 0.05

The proportion was more in cases than controls for Ranges 1 and 2; and less in cases than controls in Range 6.

For Group B: Statistically significant difference in proportions between cases and controls was recorded only in Range 2; cases more than controls. t = 4.375. df 112.

p< 0.001. The tendency in the other ranges below Range 6 (>100/min) was for cases to be more than controls. In Range 6 the tendency was for controls to be more than cases in number.

Table 4. MATCHED PAIRS OF CASES AND CONTROLS BY HEART RATE BELOW OR ABOVE AVERAGE

	Control With HR	Control With HR	McNemar's test
Group A	Below Average	Above Average	p value
Cases HR below Av.	7	19	X = 14.5. df 1
Cases HR above Av.	1	13	p<0.001. OR 5.5
Group B			
Cases HR below Av.	8	25	X = 20.3 df 1
Cases HR above Av.	1	24	p<0.001. OR 15.0

Discussion

Stroke is a common clinical condition encountered the world over. Its major risk factors include hypertension and diabetes mellitus. Minor risk factors consist of obesity, anaemia, dehydration, congestive cardiac failure, sickle cell disease and extra-cranial arterial disease [10]. Others are oral contraceptives [11], anti-hypertensive treatment in elderly patients [12], migraine [13], cigarette smoking, hyperlipidaemia, physical inactivity, age, prior stroke, coronary heart disease, left ventricular hypertrophy [14], polycythaemia, thrombocytopaenia, hyperviscousity syndrome, paroxysmal nocturnal haemoglobinuria [15], high R wave appearance on electrocardiogram and hypertensive end organ effect even if blood pressure is normal from medication [16]. Also included are some connective tissue diseases, season, leukaemia, pregnancy [17], alcohol abuse [18], male gender, snoring and sleep apnoea [19]. So are cardiac rhythm abnormalities especially atrial fibrillation [20,21]. With advances in knowledge, newer risk factors are emerging. These include raised blood homocysteine levels, anti-phospholipid antibodies and specific genetic factors [22]. Bradycardia or low heart rate is not usually considered a risk factor. Although a few studies have reported an association between bradycardia and stroke [6,7], only one report was encountered attributing the cerebral infarction to bradycardia [23].

The results of this study show that heart rate is significantly lower in stroke patients than in controls who have similar background diseases. (See Tables 1, 2, 3, and 4). This is an attempt to formally explore the importance of heart rate as a prognostic factor and potential therapeutic target. Despite suggestive evidence, this is said to be unaccepted as yet or formally explored [4]. Higher resting heart rate is known to be associated with all-cause and cardiovascular mortality among both the general population and those with hypertension or left ventricular dysfunction [24]. The same applies to acute coronary syndromes [25]. For coronary artery disease, the beneficial effects of beta blockers is said to be related to the reduction in heart rate [26]; as lowering heart rate reduces oxygen demand by reducing contractility [27]. For congestive cardiac failure, heart rate reduction by beta blockers lowers oxygen requirement for non-mechanical work; thereby increasing mechanical efficiency [28]. It must be stated however that heart rate reduction is not the only mechanism by which beta blocker therapy benefits these categories of patients [29].

In looking at the association between stroke and reduced heart rate, there is a tendency to postulate that Cushing's reflex resulting from increased intra-cranial pressure in the acute phase of stroke is responsible. However intra-cerebral haemorrhage, the variety of stroke likely to be associated with increased intra-cranial pressure [30] and hence Cushing's reflex constitutes only about 10% to 15% of all strokes [31]. This makes that position unlikely to be the rule. To remove the effect of this possible confounder in this study, patients who had recovered from acute stroke with or without residual disability, and were being followed up in the out-patient clinic were considered separately (group B). Having recovered from the acute phase, any raised intra-cranial pressure and hence Cushing's reflex would have disappeared. These patients (group B) still had significantly lower heart rates than their controls (Tables 2, 3 and 4). It is important to point out that heart rate or pulse rate vary with physiological state, which is bound to fluctuate over a given period. Although it would be difficult to control for everything, one would expect that since cases and controls were examined in the same setting over the same time, most of the extraneous factors would have been taken care of.

Not withstanding any such draw back (patients' state of mind, stress level and personality type), the findings of our study are interesting and could at least in part explain the increased stroke rates in hypertensives (especially the aged) treated with beta blockers [32,33,34,35]. Most (about 70%) of strokes are ischaemic and arise from arterial thrombo-embolism [31]. Patients with major risk factors for stroke more often than not have athero and arteriosclerosis. This presents an injured endothelial surface which is one of the primary influences predisposing to thrombus formation. This contributes to thrombogenesis when plaques on such surfaces rupture, ulcerate or erode exposing highly thrombogenic surfaces which allow platelets to adhere and become activated. These platelet aggregates may then discharge debris into the blood stream producing micro-emboli that cause stroke [36]. When the heart rate is slow as in the aged, with beta blocker therapy or during sleep, blood flow becomes sluggish. Stasis is easily created and this disrupts normal laminar flow of blood [37]. This pattern of flow (laminar), ensures that platelets flow centrally in the middle of the vessel. Turbulence of blood flow exists in narrow vessels (as can result from atherosclerosis of ageing and major risk factors of stroke), sharp turns and bifurcation or ulcerated plaques [38]. The eddy current created at these points causes blood to flow with much greater resistance. This worsens stasis that gives time for platelets to stick to damaged vessel wall and one another. They then upon aggregation, release their vaso-active contents which trigger the series of activities leading to thrombus formation. When thrombi are of sufficient size, they can cause vascular occlusion with cerebral ischaemia and stroke as consequences [39]. The increased plasma fibrinogen level in many patients at risk for cerebrovascular disease [40], and reduced fibrinolytic activity in these patients with atherosclerosis [41] ensures that any such thrombi formed do not dissolve. Embolisation following dislodgement caused by surge in heart rate and blood pressure on rising or during rapid eye movement of sleep can also lead to ischemic stroke. Ischaemic vascular disorders are known to occur more on rising [42].The foregoing could therefore be the explanation or partly thereof of beta blocker therapy (which reduces heart rate) increasing stroke rates especially in the elderly; and for an increased tendency to stroke in at risk individuals with lower than normal heart rates.

Various factors are known to predispose individuals to stroke. While some are major, others are relatively minor. Cerebrovascular disease is one area where aetiological factors overlap tremendously. It is a well recognized fact that the epidemiology of every chronic disease (like stroke) is determined by a complex interplay of contributory factors. While some are of aetiological importance, others operate as indirect markers of hitherto unknown variables [43]. For instance hypertension, diabetes mellitus, obesity [10], hypercholesterolaemia [14] and snoring [19] are risk factors in their own rights. It is however important to note that the obese patient is very likely to be hypertensive, diabetic, hypercholesterolaemic and to snore at night. One could then imagine how difficult it would be controlling for confounders and contaminants in studies of aetiological factors of stroke. Irrespective of the aetiological factors, there are triggering mechanisms, increasing knowledge of which helps to plan preventive and curative treatment.

Low heart rate or bradycardia in extreme cases is one condition which in our view point has a role to play in the aetio-pathogenesis of stroke. Heart rate is one human variable that is highly dependent on time, place and person. Controlling for it to elucidate its proper role in stroke has proved daunting. However a few facts and experiences are germane in positing this factor appropriately. Incidence of stroke rises with age [14]. Heart rate decreases with age [14, 44]. Stroke occurs frequently with inactivity [14]. The heart rate would be expectedly lower in physical inactivity. Stroke rates are highest during sleep [42]. The heart rate is low at these times. Thrombosis is a feature of sluggish circulation or stasis [37]. Bradycardia or low heart rate makes for sluggish circulation. Recently it was found that hypertensive patients treated with beta blockers (which reduce heart rate) had higher stroke rates than those treated with calcium channel blockers (those that either increase or are neutral to heart rate) [32]. One of the authors (BNO) has encountered some anecdotal cases of cerebrovascular disease where there was sinus bradycardia and no major risk factor for stroke (Unpublished personal experience). The implication of this therefore is that persons who by virtue of major or minor risk factors are at risk for cerebrovascular disease would benefit highly from anti-platelet drugs if their heart rates are below average. This category of patients should benefit from use of such drugs in primary prevention and more from secondary prevention of stroke. Before now, benefits from anti-platelet drugs in primary prevention have not been consistently shown [45]. This may have to do with inclusion of all ranges of heart rate in such studies. Alternatively, calcium entry blockers known to increase heart rate may be the preferred regimen if such patients are hypertensive in addition.

The question may then be asked. Is there an optimal heart rate? Studies have shown a continuous increase in cardiovascular risk with increasing heart rate [46, 47]; and one for heart rates below 60 per minute [48]. Such an optimum in our view should be around 70 per minute [9], but would be expected to differ from one individual to the other depending on the underlying physiological or pathophysiological status. For stroke however, it would appear that the lower the heart rate among other risk factors, the greater the chances of developing the condition. A larger scale study (to increase the sample size) and utilizing modern neuro-imaging techniques to confirm clinical diagnosis of stroke is called for to put the subject in a clearer perspective.

References

[1] Schoenberg BS. Neurologic disease in the elderly: Epidemiologic considerations. *Seminar in Neurology*. 1981;1(1): 5 – 11.

[2] Barnejee TK, Roy MK, Bhoi KK. Is stroke increasing in India – Preventive measures that need to be implimented. *J. Indian Med. Assoc.* 2005; 103(3): 162, 164, 166. passim.

[3] Komolafe MA, Ogunlade O, Komolafe EO. Stroke mortality in a Teaching Hospital in South Western Nigeria. (Letters). *Afr. J. Neurol. Sc.* 2006; 25(2): 75 - 77.

[4] Fox K, Borer JS, Camm JA, Danchin N, Ferrari R, Lopez Sendon JL, Tardif JC, Tarazzi L, Tendera M. for the Heart Rate Working Group. Resting Heart Rate in Cardiovascular Disease. *J. Am. Coll. Cardiol.* 2007; 50(9): 823 – 830.

[5] Bangalore S, Messerli FH, Kostis JB, Pepine CJ. Cardiovascular protection using beta blockers. *J. Am. Coll. Cardiol.* 2007; 50(7): 563 – 572.

[6] O'Brien MT, Pallet PJ. The major cardiovascular conditions associated with stroke (sinus bradycardia and heart block). In: MT O'Brien, PJ Pallet (Eds). Total Care of the Stroke Patient. 1st edition. 1978. Little Brown and Co. Boston. p. 188 – 199.

[7] Ike VO, Nwosu MC, Nwabueze AC. The epidemiology of stroke in Nigerians. A study of 328 cases. *Trop. Card.* 1988; 14(54): 63 – 67.

[8] Chiu EH, Tan TY, Chang KC, Liou CW. Risk factors for ischaemic stroke: electrocardiographic findings. *Acta Neurol.* Taiwan. 2006; 15(4): 232 – 236.

[9] Ganong WF. Origin of the heart beat and the electrical activity of the heart. In: WF Ganong (Ed). Review of Medical Physiology. 16th edition. 1993. Appleton and Lange. London. Sydney. Toronto. Mexico. New Delhi. Tokyo. Singapore. Rio de Janeiro. New Jersey. P. 494 – 504.

[10] Osuntokun BO. Stroke in the Africans. *Afr. J. Med. Med. Sc.* 1977; 6: 39 – 53.

[11] Fortney JA, Harper JM, Potts M. Oral contraceptives and life expectancy. *Stud. Fam. Plan.* 1986; 17(3): 117 – 125.

[12] Jansen PA, Schele BP, Mayboom RH, Gribnau FW. Antihypertensive treatment as possible cause of stroke in the elderly. *Age – ageing*. 1986; 15(3): 129 – 138.

[13] Welch KM, Levine SR, Migraine related stroke in the context of international Headache Society Classification of Head pain. *Arch. Neurol.* 1990; 47(4): 458 – 462.

[14] Aronow WS. Risk factors for geriatric stroke. Identification and follow up. *Geriatrics.* 1990; 45(9): 37 – 40, 43 – 44.

[15] Warlow C. Cerebrovascular diseases. Pathogenesis, diagnosis and complications. In: RAC Hughes and B. Matthews (Eds). Disorders of the Nervous System (II) 1980. Medical Education International Ltd. Oxford, England. P. 1991 – 1994.

[16] Shimamota T, Komachi Y, Inada H, Doi M, Iso H, Sato S, Kitamura A, Iida M, Konishi M, Nakanishi N, Terao A, Naito Y, Kojima S. Trends in coronary heart disease and stroke and their risk factors in Japan. *Circ.* 1989; 79(3): 503 – 515.

[17] Housely E. Definition of risk factors in stroke. In. FJ Gillingham, C Maudsley, AE Williams (Eds). Stroke. Proceedings of the 9th Pfizer International Symposium. 1976. Churchill Livingstone. Edinburgh. London. New York. P. 251 – 262.

[18] Marmot MG, Poulter MR. Primary prevention of stroke. Lancet 1992; 339: 344 – 347.

[19] Palomaki H, Partinen M, Erkinjuntti T, Kaste M. Snoring, sleep apnoea syndrome and stroke. *Neurol.* 1992; 42(7 Supp 6): 75 – 82 (S).

[20] Wollff PA, Kannel WB, Verter J. Current status of risk factors for stroke. *Neurol. Clin.* 1983; 1: 317 – 343.

[21] Lip GY, Tse HF. Management of atrial fibrillation. Lancet 2007; 370(9581): 604 – 618.

[22] Albert GW, Alberts MJ, Broderick JP, Lyden PD, Sacco RL. Recent advances in stroke management. *J. Stroke Cerebrovasc. Dis.* 2000; 9(3): 95 – 105.

[23] Hayabuchi Y, Matsoka S, Nii M, Suzuya H, Kuroda Y. Cerebral infarction in a patient with congenital complete heart block. *Clin. Cardiol.* 1998; 21(4): 302 – 303.

[24] Palatini P, Benetos A, Julius S. Impact of increased heart rate on clinical outcomes in hypertension: implications for antihypertensive drug therapy. *Drugs.* 2006; 66: 133 – 144.

[25] Kovar D, Cannon CP, Bentley JH, Charlesworth A, Rogers WJ. Does initial and delayed heart rate predict mortality in patients with acute coronary syndrome? *Clin. Cardiol.* 2004; 27: 80 – 86.

[26] Kjekshus JK. Importance of heart rate in determining beta blocker efficacy in acute and long term acute myocardial infarction intervention trials. *Am. J. Cardiol.* 1986; 57: 43 F – 49F.

[27] Tanaka N, Nozawa T, Yasumura T, Futaki S, Hiramori K, Suga H. Heart rate proportional oxygen consumption for constant cardiac work in dog heart. *Jpn. J. Physiol.* 1990; 40: 503 521.

[28] Yamakawa H, Takeuchi M, Takaoka H, Hata K, Mori M, Yokoyama M. Negative chronotropic effect of beta blockade therapy reduces myocardial oxygen expenditure for non-mechanical work. *Circulation.* 1996; 94: 340 – 345.

[29] Gullestad L, Wikstrand J, Deedwania P. What resting heart rate should one aim for when treating patients with heart failure with a beta blocker? Experience from the Metoprolol Controlled Release/Extended Release randomized intervention trial in chronic heart failure. (MERIT-HF). *J. Am. Coll. Cardiol.* 2005; 45: 252 – 259.

[30] Danesi MA. Management of high blood pressure in acute stroke. *Niger. Med. J.* 1995; 28(3): 134 – 139.

[31] Kaplan NM. Primary Hypertension: Natural History, Special Populations and Evaluation. In: NM Kaplan (Ed). Clinical Hypertension. 6th Edition. William and Wilkins. Baltimore. USA. 1994. P. 109 – 143.

[32] Dahlof B, Sever PS, Poulter NR. Prevention of cardiovascular events with an antihypertensive regimen of amlodipine adding perindopril as required versus atenolol adding bendroflumethiazide as required in the Anglo-Scandinavian Cardiac Outcomes trial blood pressure lowering arm (ASCOT – BPLA): a multi centre randomized controlled trials. *Lancet.* 2005; 366: 895 – 906.

[33] Bradley HA, Wiysonge CS, Volmink JA, Mayosi BM, Opie LH. How strong is the systemic evidence for use of a beta blocker as first line therapy for hypertension? Systemic review and meta analysis. *J. Hypertens.* 2006; 24: 2131 – 2141.

[34] Khan M, McAlister FA. Re-examining the efficacy of beta blockers for the treatment of hypertension: a meta analysis. *CMAJ.* 2006;174: 1737 – 1742.

[35] Lindholm LH, Calberg B, Samuelsson O. Should beta blockers remain first choice in the treatment of primary hypertension? A meta analysis. *Lancet* 2005; 366: 1545 – 1553.

[36] Schoen FJ. Blood vessels. In: V Kumar, AK Abass, N Fausto (Eds). Robbins and Contran Pathological Basis of Disease with Illustrations by JA Perkins. 7th edition. 2005. Elsevier and Saunders. Philadelphia Pennsylvania. P.511 – 554.

[37] Mitchel RN. Haemodynamic Disorders, Thromboembolic disease and shock. Ibid. 36. p. 161 – 169.

[38] Guyton AC, Hall JE. Overview of the Circulation: Medical Physics of Pressure, Flow and Resistance. In: AC Guyton, JE Hall (Eds). Text-book of Medical Physiology. 9th edition. WB Saunders Co. Philadelphia, London, Toronto, Montreal, Sydney, Tokyo. P. 161 -169.

[39] Wekssler BB. Platelet function and anti-platelet agents. In: HJM Barnett, JB Mohr, BM Stein, FM Yatsu (Eds). Stroke: Pathology, Diagnosis and Management. 3rd edition. 1998. Churchill Livingstone. New York, Philadelphia, Edinburgh, London, Toronto, Montreal, Sydney, Tokyo. P. 1041 – 1059.

[40] Shankar A, Wang JJ, Rochtina E, Mitchell P. Positive Association between plasma fibrinogen level and incident hypertension among men. Population based cohort study. *Hypertension.* 2006; 48: 1043 – 1049.

[41] Masumeci V, Rosa S, Caruso AI, Zuppi C, Zappacosta B, Tutinelli F. Abnormal diurnal changes in in-vivo platelet activation in patients with atherosclerotic disease. *Atheroscl.* 1986; 60: 231 – 236.

[42] Wroe SJ, Sandercock P, Bamford T, Dennis M, Slattery J, Warlow C. Diurnal variation in incidence of stroke: Oxfordshire Community Stroke Projects. BMJ. 1992; 304(6820): 155 – 157.

[43] Thelle D. Prevention of cardiovascular diseases – a scientific dilemma (Leader). Scand. *Cardiovasc. J.* 2000; 34: 103 – 105.

[44] Caird EI. Medicine inold age. In: DJ Weatherall, JGG Ledingham, DA Warell (Eds). Oxford Text-book of Medicine. 1st edition. 1984. Oxford University Press. Oxford. p. 25.3 – 25.11.

[45] Hennekens CH, Burring JE, Sandercock P. Aspirin and other anti-platelet drugs in the secondary and primary prevention of cardiovascular diseases. *Circulation.* 1989; 80(4): 749 – 756.

[46] Jouven X, Empana JP, Schwartz M, Denos M, Courbon D, Ducimetiere P. Heart rate profile during exercise as a predictor of sudden death. *N. Eng. J. Med.* 2005; 352: 1951 – 1958.

[47] Diaz A, Bourassa MG, Guertin MC, Tardiff JC. Long term prognostic value of resting heart rate in patients with suspected or proven coronary artery disease. *Eur. Heart J.* 2005; 26: 967 – 974.

[48] Lee KL, Wrodlief LH, Topol EJ. Predictors of 30 day mortality in the era of reperfusion for acute myocardial infarction: results from an international trial of 41,021 patients. *Circulation.* 1995; 91: 1659 – 1668.

In: Hypertension, Heredity and Stroke
Editor: Cristina Moratinos and Bruno Cardenas
ISBN 978-1-60741-496-4

Chapter 7

Standards and Pitfalls Regarding the SHR Model in Genetic Hypertension and Stroke

***Hiroshi Yao*[1] *and Toru Nabika*[2]**
[1] Center for Emotional and Behavioral Disorders,
National Hospital Organization Hizen Psychiatric Center, Saga, Japan
[2] Department of Functional Pathology, School of Medicine,
Shimane University, Izumo, Japan

1. Introduction

Spontaneously hypertensive rats (SHR) was developed by Okamoto and Aoki (1963) [1] by selective inbreedings from the Wistar-Kyoto rats (WKY). SHR are relevant to stroke research and are used widely for studies of hypertension-related cerebraovascular complications. However, one of the most annoying problems with using SHR in stroke research is that SHR or its normotensive control WKY from different sources are genetically heterogeneous. SHR/Izm have emerged as a prototype of SHR, which are derived from original SHR. The SHRSP was originally established from the A substrain of the SHR, and two other substrains of SHR, the B and C substrains, are stroke resistant. B substrain corresponds to SHR/Izm.

We have established a focal ischemia model utilizing the laser system (photothrombotic distal middle cerebral artery [MCA] occlusion and YAG laser induced reperfusion) [2]. Photothrombotic occlusion of distal MCA in SHR provides a simple and reproducible model of stroke or focal ischemia. A congenic strategy using inbred rat strains that display genetic hypertension (i.e., SHR) is a powerful method by which to examine the effects of polygenic traits on the stroke phenotype [3]. Recently, we examined the effects of the congenic removal of a blood pressure quantitative trait locus (QTL) on stroke phenotype (i.e., infarct volume after MCA occlusion [MCAO]) [4]. Based on this experience, we would like to comment on the standards and pitfalls of stroke models in the research on genetic hypertension and stroke.

2. The Stroke Model

In SHR, both blood pressure levels and global ischemia-induced deterioration of brain metabolism (i.e., increased lactate and decreased ATP) progress with age, and reaches a plateau at the age of 5 months [5]. Mori et al. [6] compared survival rates, body weight, and systolic blood pressures (the tail-cuff method) between male WKY and SHR. Blood pressure of SHR rises between 1 and 5 months, and remained constant until 22 months. Body weight of SHR was constant after 5 months. Survival rate of male SHR declines steeply after 15 months of age. Based on these observations, we recommend to use SHR at 5 to 7 months for adult models of focal ischemia.

We usually purchase SHR/Izm from a commercial vendor (Japan SLC) at age of 3 months and maintain at least 2 months in our laboratory. Rats are fed regular rat chow (CLEA rodent diet CE-2, containing 25% protein, Na^+ 2.6 mg/g pellet, and K^+ 10.6 mg/g pellet) and tap water ad libitum.

Details of our focal ischemia model were described previously [2, 7, 8]. Briefly, rats were anesthetized with halothane (3% for induction, 1.5% during the surgical preparation with a face mask, 0.75% after intubation, and 0.5% for maintenance) in a mixture of 70% nitrous oxide and 30% oxygen. The right femoral artery and vein were cannulated using PE 50 tubing.

Table 1. Physiological variables and infarct size

BW	(g)	359 ± 15
MABP	(mmHg)	176 ± 11
Temp head	(℃)	36.5 ± 0.2
Temp rectum	(℃)	37.2 ± 0.3
Arterial blood gases		
pCO_2	(mmHg)	38.4 ± 2.8
pO_2	(mmHg)	107 ± 12
pH		7.42 ± 0.02
Blood glucose	(mmol/L)	8.22 ± 1.23
Plasma electrolytes		
Na	(mmol/L)	139 ± 2
K	(mmol/L)	3.9 ± 0.2
iCa	(mmol/L)	1.23 ± 0.05
Infarct volume	(mm^3)	87 ± 20

Values are mean±S.D. (n=16).

BW, body weight; MABP, mean arterial blood pressure.

The rats were endotracheally intubated with PE 240 tubing, pancuronium bromide (an initial dose of 0.3 mg followed by 0.1 mg every 30 min) was intravenously injected, and the rats were mechanically ventilated. Mean arterial blood pressure was continuously monitored. Rats were mounted on a stereotaxic head holder in the prone position, and a burr hole 3 mm in diameter was made 1 mm rostral to the anterior junction of the zygoma and squamosal bone under an operating microscope (OPMI 111, Carl Zeiss), revealing the distal segment of the MCA.

The anatomy of distal MCA was recorded by drawing under the operating microscope (X20) and was classified into 3 categories (simple/regular/complicated) as previously described [8]. A krypton laser operating at 568 nm (643-Y-A01, Melles Griot Inc.) was used to irradiate the distal MCA at a power of 20 mW for 4 min. The photosensitizing dye rose bengal (15 mg/mL in 0.9% saline; Wako) was administered intravenously to a body dose of 20 mg/kg over 90 sec starting simultaneously with 4 min of laser irradiation. The irradiated MCA was consistently occluded within 3 min. Three days or 24 hours after ischemic insult, the infarct volume was determined on TTC-stained sections.

Table 2. Reproducibility of Infarct Size

			Infarct Volume, mm^3				
Surgeon	Strain	Sex	Mean	±	S.D.	n	C.V.
Y-1	SHR/Kyushu	M	85	±	17	6	21
	Sprague-Dawley	M	12	±	2	4	19
Y-2	SHR/Kyushu	M	93	±	23	8	25
T-1	SHR/Kyushu	M	95	±	20	12	22
T-2	SHR/Kyushu	M	116	±	27	8	23
T-3	SHR/Kyushu	F	58	±	14	8	25
	SHR/Kyushu*	F	88	±	16	8	18
C-1	SHR/Kyushu	M	84	±	12	8	14
	SHR/Izm	M	62	±	11	10	17
	SHR/Kyushu	F	59	±	9	8	16
	SHR/Izm	F	35	±	8	5	23
	WKY/Izm	M	23	±	4	6	16
C-2	SHR/Izm	M	63	±	12	7	19
	SHR/Izm	M	56	±	6	7	11
O	SHR/Kyushu	M	70	±	16	5	22
F	SHR/Kyushu	F	61	±	16	5	27
	SHR/Kyushu	F	55	±	16	5	29
K-1	SHR/Kyushu	M	115	±	38	10	33
K-2	SHR/Kyushu	M	101	±	18	7	18
S	SHR/Kyushu	M	84	±	11	9	13
Y-3	SHR/Kyushu	M	100	±	31	5	31
	SHRSP/Izm	M	97	±	25	6	26
Y-4	SHR/Kyushu	M	82	±	18	6	22

Reprinted in modified form from Yao H, et al. (*Stroke* 2003;**34**:2716-2721)
Coefficient of variation (C.V.) = S.D./mean.
M, male; F, female; *Female aged SHR/Kyushu.

Anesthesia should be without an intrinsic neuroprotective activity. Physiological monitoring such as blood pressure, blood gases, glucose, and brain temperature is essential to maintain the animals properly. Brain temperature is a critical variable to be monitored and maintained as constant as possible throughout the experiment. *Table 1* shows physiological variables and infarct volume in our recent experiment of 16 sequential SHR/Izm. Reproducibility of infarct size in our stroke model is demonstrated in *Table 2* [2].

3. Sex Differences in Experimental Stroke

The infarct size after MCAO is significantly smaller in female SHR compared with male counterpart [8]. This smaller infarct size of female SHR could be due to lower blood pressure levels of female SHR, or due to neuroprotective effects of sex steroids. The infarct volume produced 4 weeks after ovariectomy was significantly increased in female SHR [9]. The increased infarct size in ovariectomized female SHR was similar to that of male SHR. Estradiol replacement (200μg/kg of estradiol valerate, subcutaneously injected once a week) after ovariectomy attenuated the infarction. Because blood pressure was not affected by ovariectomy or estradiol replacement, estrogen was considered to contribute to the differences in infarct volume between male and female SHR.

Alkayed et al. [10] demonstrated that both cortical and striatal infarct sizes were smaller in female rats compared with those in ovaiectomized female and male rats. Ovarientomy increased and physiologically relevant amounts of 17β-estradiol attenuated infarct size. Several studies indicated that estrogen must be administered chronically before ischemic insults to be effective in ovariectomized female rats [11, 12]. In contrast, Carswell et al. [13] observed that female SHRSP with high levels of estrogen (proestrus) showed smaller infarction after MCAO than those with low levels of estrogen (metestrus) during the 4-day rat estrus cycle. The protective effect of physiological doses of estrogen did not appear to be the result of improved cerebral blood flow (CBF) after MCAO. Estrogen act as potent antioxidants and inhibit oxidative damage in cerebral ischemia and reperfusion [12]. Estrogens may protect against ischemic injury through genomic mechanisms, because the actions of estradiol are often slow and required pretreatment. Estradiol promoted cell survival in focal ischemia via the antiapoptotic protein, Bcl-2, and the action of estradiol was suggested to be mediated through estrogen receptorβ [14, 15].

4. Age-Related Vulnerability

We investigated age-related vulnerability to cerebral ischemia found in global ischemia [16] in the context of focal ischemia or stroke. Infarct volume of aged female SHR produced by photothrombotic distal MCAO was significantly larger than that of adult SHR (89±16 mm^3 vs. 58±14 mm^3) [17]. Increased infarct size was demonstrated in aged Wistar rats compared with yonger rats [18, 19]. In these studies, the regional CBF determined with laser-Doppler flowmetry or the hydrogen clearance method, respectively, was not different between the two age groups. Therefore, factors other than blood flow may be responsible for age-related vulnerability to focal ischemia or brain infarction. Alkayed et al. [20] and Dubal and Wise [21] reported that both estrogen and progensterone treatment reduced cortical infarct in reproductively senescent female Wistar rats (16-months old) or in middle-aged female Sprague-Dawley rats (9- to 12-months old). These results suggest that decreased hormones in reproductively inactive female rats deteriorate ischemic injury. In our experiment, however, plasma levels of 17β-estradiol and progesterone determined with radioimmunoassay were not different between the two age groups [17]. Thus, we conclude that age-related vulnerability found in female SHR is not the result of decreased sex hormones in aged rats.

5. Distal MCA Patterns

The anatomy of distal MCA was observed in 85 male SHR/Kyushu, 127 Sprague-Dawley rats, and 42 Wistar rats, and was classified into 8 branching patterns and then 3 categories (simple/ regular/ complicated) [8]. We found that about half of distal MCA in SHR were simple, and only a small number of SHR had a complicated artery. Infarct volume of SHR with simple Y-shaped MCA was smaller than that of the regular pattern. This phenomenon was reproducible as exemplified by a recent experiment in sequential 16 SHR/Izm: 73.6±18.3 mm^3 vs. 96.6±14.7 mm^3 ($p=0.014$) in rats with simple and regular distal MCA, respectively. Menzies et al. [22] failed to find any relationship between the anatomical pattern of MCA and the surface size of the brain infarction in Sprague-Dawley rats. The reason for the discrepancy between these two studies is not clear, but our data indicate an important caveat to stroke genetics studies as well as pharmacoprotection studies.

6. Substrain Differences

We examined substrain differences between SHR/Kyushu and SHR/Izm. SHR/Kyushu was derived from the F20 generation of original SHR, and have been maintained in Kyushu University Animal Center under specific pathogen free conditions for more than 30 years [23]. Mean arterial blood pressure was 183±2 (S.D.) mmHg in male SHR/Kyushu, 180±7 mmHg in male SHR/Izm, 161±5 mmHg in female SHR/Kyushu, and 155±5 mmHg in female SHR/Izm [8]. Brain infarction produced by distal MCAO was larger in SHR/Kyushu compared with SHR/Izm in both male and female rats. Because blood pressure levels were the same between the two substrains, factors other than hypertension probably account for different lesion size. We also compared the mean infarct volume of male SHRSP/Izm with that of SHR/Kyushu at 5- to 6-months old [17]. Body weight of SHRSP/Izm was significantly less than that of SHR/Kyushu, and mean arterial blood pressure was higher in SHRSP/Izm by about 40 mmHg compared with that in SHR/Kyushu. Nonetheless, infarct volumes were almost the same between SHRSP/Izm and SHR/Kyushu. Again presumed genetic factors other than the blood pressure level appeared to contribute to different infarct size or stroke sensitivity among substrains of SHR/Izm.

7. Congenic Removal of a QTL for Blood Pressure

Stroke is a disease of complex, multifactorial, and polygenic trait caused by an interaction between genetics and environmental factors. Brain infarction is the most common type of stroke. However, the heterogeneity of risk factors and distinct subtype of brain infarction in human ischemic stroke complicates the investigation into genetic aspect of stroke. The single largest cause of stroke is hypertension, which is itself complex, polygenic trait. Therefore, it is immensely advantageous to study rodent models.

A few studies using genome-wide scanning strategy identified quantitative trait loci (QTL), a large chromosomal region which contains a gene or number of genes, responsible for the quantitative trait for susceptibility to stroke. Rubattu et al. [24] demonstrated three QTL for the latency to stroke in the SHR×SHRSP/Hd cross. Three QTL were mapped to chromosome 1, 4, and 5, and the chromosome 5 locus, localized in close proximity to the gene encoding atrial natriuretic factor, protected from stroke in the hypertensive rats. The number of days necessary to develop stroke (stroke proneness) was blood pressure independent. With regard to the extent of ischemic damage after MCAO (stroke sensitivity), Jeffs et al. [25] found a highly significant QTL on rat chromosome 5, using SHRSP/Gla×WKY cross. The microsatellite marker in the center of this QTL was again the gene encoding atrial natriuretic factor.

The discovery of QTL is the first step of the ultimate goal of "yet unknown" gene identification. The QTL has to be confirmed, usually by the congenic strategy. A congenic strain is one that has a region of its genome selectively replaced by the same region from another strain. With this strategy, Rubattu et al.[26] showed that a QTL on rat chromosome 1 derived from an SHR background introgressed into the SHRSP background influenced stroke proneness without affecting blood pressure levels. This congenic strategy must be followed by the procedure of fine genetic substitution mapping to narrow down the existing QTL to 1 cM or less, a requisite size at which positional cloning is feasible.

We investigated the effects of congenic removal of the blood pressure QTL from SHRSP/Izm on the infarct size after MCAO and assessed the contribution of hypertension on the stroke vulnerability [4]. The congenic removal of a QTL for blood pressure substantially reduced infarct size by 36%, while it decreased blood pressure by 12% in adult rats. In young adult rats (10-12 week old), both blood pressure and infarct size were not different between SHRSP/Izm and the congenic rats (SHRSPwch1.0). These results indicated that the absence of one of the blood pressure QTLs protected SHRSP against brain infarction principally through decreasing blood pressure. CBF determined at collaterally-perfused cortex with laser-Doppler flowmetry was significantly greater in adult SHRSPwch1.0 compared with CBF in adult SHRSP/Izm. Therefore, the mechanism of decreased infarct size in the congenic rats was considered to be caused by increased collateral CBF due to chronic effects of lowering blood pressure.

8. Cerebral Blood Flow

With regard to CBF, the golden standard for focal ischemia models is 3-dimensional autoradiography [27]. Laser-Doppler flowmetry is an easy method, and is commonly used in small animals. However, in the studies of focal ischemia, one-point CBF measurement with laser-Doppler flowmetry may show no significant (a false negative) difference in CBF after MCAO between the control and the genetically-engineered groups. 2-demensional cortical CBF mapping is possible with laser Doppler perfusion imaging (Moor Instruments, Inc.): a sophisticated and robust image registration method was developed by Riyamongkol et al. with this 2-demensional mapping [28]. This system, however, needs an expensive set-up.

We determined CBF with the laser-Doppler flowmetry "scanning" method as previously described [2, 4]. Briefly, a laser-Doppler flowmetry probe was laterally scanned, and CBF of the distal MCA territory was measured at five points (2 mm posterior and 2.0, 2.5, 3.0, 3.5, and 4.0 mm lateral to the bregma). Five CBF values in one rat were transformed to an area under curve according to the trapezoidal rule. As shown in Fig. 4 of our paper [4], none of the five one-point measurements find significant differences between SHRSP/Izm and the congenic rats, whereas the scanning method and area under curve revealed a clear difference in CBF between the two groups. In studies of focal ischemia, one-point CBF measurement with laser-Doppler flowmetry frequently showed no significant differences between the groups because of type II error. If we had done one-point measurement, for example at 4 mm lateral to the bregma, the conclusion would be that there is no significant difference in CBF after MCAO between SHRSP and SHRSPwch1.0, suggesting some unknown "genetic" effects on infarct size.

9. Reperfusion Injury

In genetic studies concerning experimental stroke, to make the supposition that the genetic factor(s) being studied play a role in the pathophysiology of reperfusion requires reperfusion stroke models. It is not enough, however, merely for reperfusion to occur as a requirement to satisfy such a model. It's obvious that not all ischemic injury after reperfusion is reperfusion injury. As evidenced by the definition of reperfusion injury as "when the condition of ischemia is aggravated by the occurrence of reperfusion, more so than in the case where reperfusion does not occur (permanent occlusion)", in order to see reperfusion injury it is necessary to make a comparison with permanent occlusion [29]. There are actually very few models, however, in which it is possible to test both permanent occlusion and reperfusion. For example, while the most frequently used small animal focal ischemia model may be the intraluminal suture model, one point of view says that this model is a top of the internal carotid artery occlusion model rather than a MCAO model [30]. This model has a wide ischemia range, and because the mortality rate is high in the case of permanent occlusion, the permanent occlusion group and the reperfusion group that shared the same time lapse cannot be compared. In fact, of the "reperfusion injuries" seen in much of the research, those that exhibit real reperfusion injury are surprisingly rare. The model we have developed as mentioned above has a mortality rate of essentially 0% even with permanent occlusion, so it is possible to conduct tests with the conditions of both permanent occlusion and reperfusion in the same model, making it very useful in the condition analysis of reperfusion injury [2].

10. Statistical Power

We also need to consider sample size calculation (statistical power analysis) based on coefficient of variation (C.V. = S.D./mean) for infarct volume [31]. Duverger and MacKenzie [32] attempted to assess the variability of brain infarction induced by proximal MCAO in several rat strains. The importance of factors such as age and diabetes on the infarct volume was also examined. The infarct volume was relatively large in the Sprague-Dawley rats and with a fair variability (C.V. = 33%). In WKY, the variability was large while the infarct size was small. The Fisher-344 rats presented with a consistent and sizable infarct volume (C.V. = 20%). In contrast to these normotensive strains, proximal MCAO resulted in a considerable volume of infarction, and the variability was minimal in SHR and SHRSP. Brint et al. described an experience with focal ischemia produced by distal MCAO in three strains of rat (Wistar, Fisher-344, and SHR). Tandem occlusion of the distal MCA and ipsilateral common carotid artery in the SHR provided a surgically simple method for reproducible infarction (C.V. = 12-35%). An important measure of the practicality of the stroke model is the number of animals necessary to detect significant differences or to avoid type II (false positive) error between control and experimental (e.g., genetically-engineered) groups. Brint et al. [33] estimated that 8-31 rats are needed to detect an effect size of 25%. In our experience, an average of C.V. of infarct volume produced by distal photothrombotic MCAO in SHR was 21% (*Table 2*), indicating that 9 rats in each group is enough to exclude type II error in case of the 30% difference in infarct volume (effect size is 1.43) between the groups. We conclude that MCAO in the SHR offers a practical model in terms of requisite number of animals.

Conclusions

We described the requirements stroke models should meet and their pitfalls in the analysis of genetic factors involved in genetic hypertension and particularly stroke vulnerability in SHR. The existence of substrain differences in SHR is a difficult problem and it is essential to specify the strain to be used. Concerning stroke models, it is necessary to monitor such parameters as physiological variables including brain temperature, time of use (age), gender differences, and CBF measurement methods. In quantification of the size of the cerebral infarction, whether the variation of infarct volume is within an acceptable range should be checked with statistical power analysis. In addition, comparison of cases where reperfusion occurs and where it does not is needed in the study of reperfusion injury. Appropriate stroke models will contribute to the advancement of the analysis of the complex polygenic traits of stroke.

References

[1] Okamoto and Aoki. (1963). Development of a strain of spontaneously hypertensive rats. *Jpn Circ. J.* 27:282-293.

[2] Yao H, Sugimori H, Fukuda K, Takada J, Ooboshi H, Kitazono T, Ibayashi S, and Iida M. (2003). Photothrombotic middle cerebral artery occlusion and reperfusion laser system in spontaneously hypertensive rats. *Stroke* 34:2716-2721.

[3] Nabika T, Kobayashi Y, and Yamori Y. (2000). Congenic rats for hypertension: How useful are they for the hunting of hypertension genes? *Clin. Exp. Pharmacol. Physiol.* 27:251-256.

[4] Yao H, Cui Z-H, Masuda J, and Nabika T. (2007). Congenic removal of a QTL for blood pressure attenuates infarct size produced by middle cerebral artery occlusion in hypertensive rats. *Physiol. Genomics* 30:69-73.

[5] Tamaki K, Fujishima M, Ogata J, Nakatomi Y, Ishitsuka T, Sadoshima S, and Omae T. (1979). Effects of aging on cerebral metabolism following bilateral carotid ligation in male spontaneously hypertensive rats (SHR). *Brain Res.* 170:368-71.

[6] Mori S, Kato M, Fujishima M. (1995). Impaired maze learning and cerebral glucose utilization in aged hypertensive rats. *Hypertension* 25:545-553.

[7] Yao H, Ibayashi S, Sugimori H, Fujii K, and Fujishima M. (1996). Simplified model of krypton laser-induced thrombotic distal middle cerebral artery occlusion in spontaneously hypertensive rats. *Stroke* 27:333-336.

[8] Cai H, Yao H, Ibayashi S, Uchimura H, and Fujishima M. (1998). Photothrombotic middle cerebral artery occlusion in spontaneously hypertensive rats: influence of substrain, gender and distal middle cerebral artery patterns on infarct size. *Stroke* 29:1982-1987.

[9] Fukuda K, Yao H, Ibayashi S, Nakahara T, Uchimura H, Fujishima M. Ovariectomy exacerbates and estrogen replacement attenuates photothrombotic focal ischemic brain injury in rats. *Stroke* 31:155-60,2000.

[10] Alkayed NJ, Harukuni I, Kimes AS, London ED, Traystman RJ, Hurn PD. (1998). Gender-linked brain injury in experimental stroke. *Stroke* 29:159-65.

[11] Dubal DB, Kashon ML, Pettigrew LC, Ren JM, Finklestein SP, Rau SW, and Wise PM. (1998). Estradiol protects against ischemic injury. *J. Cereb. Blood Flow Metab*18:1253-1258.

[12] Hurn PD, Macrae IM. (2000). Estrogen as a neuroprotectant in stroke. *J. Cereb. Blood Flow Metab.* 20:631-52.

[13] Carswell1 HVO, Dominiczak2 AF, and Macrae1 IM. (2000). Estrogen status affects sensitivity to focal cerebral ischemia in stroke-prone spontaneously hypertensive rats. *Am. J. Physiol. Heart* 278:H290-H294.

[14] Dubal DB, Shughrue PJ, Wilson ME, Merchenthaler I, and Wise PM. (1999). Estradiol modulates bcl-2 in cerebral ischemia: a potential role for estrogen receptors. *J. Neurosci.*19:6385-6393.

[15] Rusa R, Alkayed NJ, Crain BJ, Traystman RJ, Kimes AS, London ED, Klaus JA, Hurn PD. (1999). 17beta-estradiol reduces stroke injury in estrogen-deficient female animals. *Stroke* 30:1665-70.

[16] Yao H, Sadoshima S, Ooboshi H, Sato Y, Uchimura H, and Fujishima M. (1991). Age-related vulnerability to cerebral ischemia in spontaneously hypertensive rats. *Stroke* 22:1414-1418.

[17] Takaba H, Fukuda K, and Yao H. (2004). Substrain differences, gender, and age of spontaneously hypertensive rats critically determine infarct size produced by distal middle cerebral artery occlusion. *Cell Mol. Neurobiol.* 24:589-598.

[18] Davis M, Mendelow AD, Perry RH, Chambers IR, and James OFW. (1995). Experimental Stroke and Neuroprotection in the Aging Rat Brain. *Stroke* 26:1072–1078.

[19] Sutherland GR, Dix GA, Auer RN, and Koehler RC. (1996). Effect of Age in Rodent Models of Focal and Forebrain Ischemia. *Stroke* 27:1663–1668.

[20] Alkayed NJ, Murphy SJ, Traystman RJ, Hurn PD, Miller VM. (2000). Neuroprotective effects of female gonadal steroids in reproductively senescent female rats. *Stroke* 31:161-8.

[21] Dubal DB and Wise PM. (2001). Neuroprotective Effects of Estradiol in Middle-Aged Female Rats. *Endocrinology* 142:43–48.

[22] Menzies SA, Hoff JT, and Betz AL. (1992). Middle cerebral artery occlusion in rats: a neurological and pathological evaluation of a reproducible model. *Neurosurgery* 31:100–107.

[23] Ogata J, Fujishima M, Morotomi Y, and Omae T. (1976). Cerebral infarction following bilateral carotid artery ligation in normotensive and spontaneously hypertensive rats: a pathological study. *Stroke* 7:54–60.

[24] Rubattu S, Volpe M, Kreutz R, Ganten U, Ganten D, and Lindpaintner K. (1996). Chromosomal mapping of quantitative trait loci contributing to stroke in a rat model of complex human disease. *Nat. Genet.* 13:429–434.

[25] Jeffs B, Clark JS, Anderson NH, Gratton J, Brosnan MJ, Gauguier D, Reid JL, Macrae IM, and Dominiczak AF. (1997). Sensitivity to cerebral ischaemic insult in a rat model of stroke is determined by a single genetic locus. *Nat. Genet.* 16:364-367.

[26] Rubattu S, Hubner N, Ganten U, Evangelista A, Stanzione R, Di Angelantonio E, Plehm R, Langanki R, Gianazza E, Sironi L, D'Amati G, and Volpe M. (2006). Reciprocal congenic lines for a major stroke QTL on rat chromosome 1. *Physiol. Genomics* 27:108-113.

[27] Zhao W, Belayev L, Ginsberg MD. (1997). Transient middle cerebral artery occlusion by intraluminal suture: II. Neurological deficits, and pixel-based correlation of histopathology with local blood flow and glucose utilization. *J. Cereb. Blood Flow Metab* 17:1281-90.

[28] Riyamongkol P, Zhao W, Liu Y, Belayev L, Busto R, and Ginsberg MD. (2002). Automated registration of laser Doppler perfusion images by an adaptive correlation approach: application to focal cerebral ischemia in the rat. *J. Neurosci. Method* 122:79-90.

[29] Yao H, Yoshii N, Akira T, Nakahara T. (2009) Reperfusion-induced temporary appearance of therapeutic window in penumbra after 2 h of photothrombotic middle cerebral artery occlusion in rats. *J. Cereb. Blood Flow Metab* 29:565-574.

[30] Kanemitsu H, Nakagomi T, Tamura A, Tsuchiya T, Kono G, and Sano K. (2002). Differences in the extent of primary ischemic damage between middle cerebral artery coagulation and intraluminal occlusion models. *J. Cereb. Blood Flow Metab.* 22:1196-204.

[31] Cohen J. The t test for means. In: Cohen J, ed. Statistical Power Analysis for the Behavioral Sciences. 2nd ed. Hillsdale, NJ: Lawrence Erlbaum Associates Inc Publishers; 1977:19–74.

[32] Duverger D and MacKenzie ET. (1998). The quantification of cerebral infarction following focal ischemia in the rat: influence of strain, arterial pressure, blood glucose concentration, and age. *J. Cereb. Blood Flow Metab.* 8:449-61.

[33] Brint S, Jacewicz M, Kiessling M, Tanabe J, and Pulsinelli W. (1988). Focal brain ischemia in the rat: methods for reproducible neocortical infarction using tandem occlusion of the distal middle cerebral and ipsilateral common carotid arteries. *J. Cereb. Blood Flow Metab.* 8:474-85.

In: Hypertension, Heredity and Stroke
Editor: Cristina Moratinos and Bruno Cardenas

ISBN 978-1-60741-496-4

Chapter 8

Hypertensive Children Have Lower Bone Mass than Normotensive Children

*Afrooz Afghani**
College of Health Sciences, TUI University, Cypress, CA, USA

Abstract

Background: The association between blood pressure (BP) and bone mineral content (BMC) has not been extensively studied in pediatrics. *Design:* Cross-sectional study. *Participants:* 187 (105 boys, 82 girls) overweight (BMI=28.7 kg/m^2) Latino children and adolescents (age=11.2 years). *Assessment of Risk Factors:* Seated systolic (SBP) and diastolic (DBP) blood pressure measured using a standard mercury sphygmomanometer. Hypertension defined by SBP or DBP above the 90th percentile for height, age, and gender. *Main Outcome Measurements:* Total body BMC measured by dual-energy x-ray absorptiometry. *Results:* There was an inverse association between SBP and BMC (r=-0.24, p=0.02) in boys; results were non-significant (p=0.27) in girls. There were no significant correlations between DBP and BMC in either boys or girls. Hypertensive boys (n=21) had lower BMC (1437 versus 1639 g; p=0.02) than normotensive boys (n=84); similarly, hypertensive girls (n=25) had lower BMC (1435 versus 1620 g; p=0.01) than normotensive girls (n=57). In post-pubertal boys (Tanner stage 4-5; n=11), inverse correlations between SBP and BMC were markedly stronger (r=-0.80, p=0.02). *Conclusion:* SBP is inversely correlated with BMC in overweight adolescents, with the strongest association observed in adolescent boys. Additionally, hypertensives have lower adjusted means of BMC than normotensives. Hypertension may be a risk factor for osteopenia in overweight children and adolescents.

* Phone: (714) 226-9840 ext. 2009, Fax: (714) 226-9845, E-mail: aafghani@tuiu.edu

Introduction

In 1980, McCarron et al. [1] published the first report of hypercalciuria in adult patients with hypertension. Since calcium is an important determinant of peak bone mass [2], it is logical to assume that urinary excretion of calcium due to hypertension would be detrimental to the growing skeleton of children and ultimately to adult bone mineral density (BMD). The link between hypertension and bone loss in adults has been previously studied but the existing evidence is inconclusive [3-5]. Tsuda et al. [3] compared the BMD of 31 hypertensive Japanese women to 14 normotensives and reported inverse correlations between lumbar spine BMD and SBP. We [4] also reported significantly lower BMC in hypertensive compared with normotensive Hispanic women living in the United States. In contrast, in a study of bone mass and bone modeling markers in hypertensive postmenopausal Spanish women, Perez-Castrillon et al. [5] found no significant association between SBP or DBP and lumbar spine bone mass.

In normotensive children, urinary calcium loss as a function of blood pressure has been observed in the upper age distribution [6]. It has also been reported that normotensive children of hypertensive adults have hypercalciuria [6-7]. Although in hypertensive rats, metabolic studies [8] have shown that hypercalciuria and subsequent hyperparathyroidism lead to reduced growth and detectable deficits in BMC, such detriments have not been observed in human beings.

In this chapter, we address the hypothesis that resting SBP and DBP will be inversely correlated with total body BMC in a large group of overweight Latino children and adolescents. In addition, examining whether hypertensive children and adolescents have lower BMC compared with normotensives is our second objective.

Methods

Study Cohort and Subject Description

A cohort of overweight Latino children with a positive family history of type 2 diabetes was established with the intention to follow longitudinally in the University of Southern California SOLAR (Study of Latino Adolescents at Risk) diabetes project.

187 children (105 boys, 82 girls) were recruited to the SOLAR project through clinics, health fairs, newspaper announcements, and word of mouth. The children were required to meet the following inclusion criteria: 1) age 8-14 years; 2) Body mass index (BMI) $\geq 85^{th}$ percentile for age and gender based on the CDC standards [9], and an initial telephone pre-screening; 3) Latino ancestry (all 4 grandparents Latino by self-report); and, 4) family history of type 2 diabetes in at least one parent, sibling, or grandparent. Children were of Mexican-American (71%), Central American (16%), or mixed Mexican-Central American (13%) heritage. Children were excluded if they had prior major illness including type 1 or type 2 diabetes, or took medications or had a condition known to influence body composition, blood pressure, or bone mass (e.g. pregnancy, glucocorticoid therapy, hyper- or hypothyroidism). The SOLAR study was approved by the Institutional Review Board, Health Science Campus

of the University of Southern California. Informed consent and assent were obtained from all parents and children, respectively.

It is noteworthy that based on inverse correlation coefficients reported in adult studies by Larijani et al. [10] between femoral neck BMD and SBP (r=-0.17) and by Tsuda et al. [3] between lumbar spine BMD and SBP (r=-0.31), we expected an effect size in the range of 0.17-0.31 which would require 64 to 213 participants. With a sample size of 187 children and an observed r value of -0.16 for SBP and BMC, we had 70 % power.

Protocol Design

Outpatient Screening Visit

Children arrived at the USC General Clinical Research Center (GCRC) at approximately 8:00 am after an overnight fast. Weight and height were measured followed by a physical examination conducted by a board certified pediatric endocrinologist. Physical examinations included Tanner staging in girls (breast stage) and in boys (pubic hair stage). Children in Tanner stages 1 or 2 were the "pre-pubertal" group; Tanner stage 3 children were defined as "pubertal"; adolescents in Tanner stages 4 or 5 were the "post-pubertal" category. A medical history was conducted including parental interview detailing family history of diabetes. Children who met the following screening criteria were invited back for further testing during an in-patient GCRC visit: a) BMI $\geq 85^{th}$ percentile for age and gender based on the CDC standards [9] based on height and weight measures at the GCRC; and, b) absence of type 1 or type 2 diabetes using the ADA guidelines [11]. Note that for the purposes of this study we used the CDC definitions for weight status in children (i.e. at risk of overweight/obesity is a BMI age/gender percentile greater than 85th). The 187 children who met the inclusion/exclusion criteria constituted the study sample.

Inpatient Visit

Of the 187 children completing the out-patient visit, all returned to the GCRC within 15 $\pm$ 10 (SD) days. Children were admitted to the GCRC in the early afternoon and then completed tests for bone mass and body composition using dual energy x-ray absorptiometry (DXA).

Detailed Methodologies

Weight, Height and Anthropometry

Height (by a wall mounted stadiometer) and weight (by a balance beam medical scale) were recorded at each visit to the nearest 0.1 cm and 0.1 kg respectively, and the average of the two measurements was used for analysis. BMI and BMI percentiles for age and gender were determined based upon established CDC normative curves using EpiInfo 2000, Version 1.1.

Bone Mineral Content and Body Composition

A whole body DXA scan was performed to determine whole body BMC (units: grams) and whole body composition (fat mass, lean mass) using a Hologic QDR 4500W (Hologic Inc., Bedford, Massachusetts). The whole body scan requires the subject to be placed supine with the arms and legs positioned according to the manufacturer's specifications. Quality control was performed daily using a phantom. The precision error (coefficient of variation for repeated measurements) was ≤1%.

Resting Blood Pressure

Blood pressure measurements were obtained from each seated subject on two separate days using a standard mercury sphygmomanometer with an appropriate size cuff. The right arm was used for all blood pressure measurements after the subject had rested quietly for 5 minutes. The same trained technician made all measurements. SBP was measured at the first appearance of a pulse sound (Korotkoff phase 1) and DBP at the disappearance of the pulse sound (Korotkoff phase 5). On each occasion, three readings of blood pressure were obtained, and the average was recorded [12]. Hypertension was defined by blood pressure above the 90th percentile for height, age, and gender [13].

Statistical Analysis

All analyses were performed using SPSS version 14.0 (SPSS Inc, Chicago, IL), with a type I error set at $p<0.05$. Descriptive statistics were performed; partial correlations were used to determine the associations of BMC with SBP, and DBP; independent t-tests and general linear models were used to compare BMC in two different groups (e.g. boys and girls or hypertensives and normotensives). A power analysis software program (Statistical Solutions, nQuery Advisor Version 3: Saugus, MA) was used for the power analysis results presented in the methods.

Results

Mean and standard deviation of participant characteristics are shown in Table 1. The youngest child was 8 years old; the oldest was 14. Mean age was 11.2 years. SBP had a range of 85 to 152 mmHg. DBP had a range of 48 to 99 mmHg. Mean of total body BMC was 1583.2 grams. Girls were significantly more mature than boys and had significantly lower DBP. There were no other significant differences between boys and girls.

Table 2 shows partial correlations between blood pressure and BMC. In the entire cohort, SBP was partially and inversely correlated with BMC (r=-0.16, p=0.03). There were no significant associations between DBP and BMC (p=0.36). In boys, SBP and BMC were partially correlated (r=-0.24, p=0.02); correlations were not significant (p=0.27) in girls. SBP and DBP were not significantly related with BMC in pre-pubertal and pubertal children (Tanner stage 1-3). In post-pubertal adolescents (Tanner stage 4-5), SBP was inversely correlated with BMC (r=-0.40, p=0.007).

Table 1. CHARACTERISTICS OF PARTICIPANTS (MEAN ± SD)

	All Subjects (n=187)	Boys (n=105)	Girls (n=82)
Age (years)	11.2 ± 1.7	11.3 ± 1.5	11.1 ± 1.8
Tanner Stage	2.3 ± 1.4	1.7 ± 1.1	2.9 ± 1.4*
Tanner 1	79 (42%)	59 (56%)	20 (25%)
Tanner 2	44 (23%)	29 (27%)	15 (18%)
Tanner 3	16 (9%)	6 (6%)	10 (12%)
Tanner 4	30 (16%)	6 (6%)	24 (29%)
Tanner 5	18 (10%)	5 (5%)	13 (16%)
Weight (kg)	66.3 ± 19.7	66.5 ± 19.1	66.0 ± 20.5
Height (cm)	150.2 ± 11.4	151.1 ± 11.1	149.2 ± 11.8
BMI (kg/m^2)	28.7 ± 5.5	28.6 ± 5.5	28.9 ± 5.5
BMI Percentile (%)	96.0 ± 2.3	95.9 ± 2.5	96.0 ± 2.2
Fat Mass (kg)	25.8 ± 10.4	25.2 ± 10.4	26.5 ± 10.4
Lean Mass (kg)	38.0 ± 10.2	38.8 ± 10.0	37.0 ± 10.4
Systolic Blood Pressure (mmHg)	110 ± 10.7	110 ± 10.1	110 ± 11.5
Diastolic Blood Pressure (mmHg)	64 ± 7.3	64 ± 7.6	62 ± 6.8†
Total Body BMC (g)	1583.2 ± 440.3	1598.6 ± 429.4	1563.6 ± 455.7

*significantly greater than boys ($p<0.0001$).
†significantly lower than boys ($p<0.05$).
BMI: Body Mass Index.
BMC: Bone Mineral Content.

Table 2. PARTIAL CORRELATIONS BETWEEN BLOOD PRESSURE AND BMC

SBP	BMC
All Subjects (n=187) ‡	-0.16†
Boys (n=105) §	-0.24†
Girls (n=82) §	-0.13
Pre- and Pubertal (n=139) (Tanner Stage 1-3) ‖	-0.04
Boys (n=94) ¶	-0.06
Girls (n=45) ¶	-0.02
Post-Pubertal (n=48) (Tanner Stage 4-5) ‖	-0.40†
Boys (n=11) ¶	-0.80†
Girls (n=37) ¶	-0.26
DBP	
All Subjects (n=187) ‡	-0.07
Boys (n=105) §	-0.15
Girls (n=82) §	0.12
Pre- and Pubertal (n=139) (Tanner Stage 1-3) ‖	-0.05
Post-Pubertal (n=48) (Tanner Stage 4-5) ‖	-0.15

*$p<0.005$.
†$p<0.05$.
‡Adjusted for gender, age, weight, height, Tanner stage.
§Adjusted for age, weight, height, Tanner stage.
‖Adjusted for gender, age, weight, height.
¶Adjusted for age, weight, height.
BMC: Bone Mineral Content.
SBP: Systolic Blood Pressure.
DBP: Diastolic Blood Pressure.

Table 3. Partial Correlations between Anthropometric Indices and BMC, SBP, DBP

Variables	BMC	SBP	DBP
WEIGHT			
All Subjects*	0.72	0.24	0.08
Boys	0.72	0.35	0.02
Girls	0.74	0.14	0.17
Pre- and Pubertal	0.78	0.28	0.06
Post-Pubertal	0.62	0.21	0.13
BMI			
All Subjects*	0.54	0.25	0.09
Boys	0.55	0.36	0.03
Girls	0.54	0.19	0.21
Pre- and Pubertal	0.60	0.29	0.08
Post-Pubertal	0.35	0.26	0.16
FAT MASS			
All Subjects*	0.55	0.23	0.09
Boys	0.56	0.37	0.06
Girls	0.59	0.16	0.15
Pre- and Pubertal	0.65	0.29	0.08
Post-Pubertal	0.35	0.29	0.16
LEAN MASS			
All Subjects*	0.81	0.21	0.04
Boys	0.81	0.28	-0.05
Girls	0.81	0.10	0.18
Pre- and Pubertal	0.85	0.23	0.01
Post-Pubertal	0.78	0.07	0.08

Bold: significant at p<0.05.
*Adjusted for gender, age, Tanner stage.
BMC: Bone Mineral Content.
SBP: Systolic Blood Pressure.
DBP: Diastolic Blood Pressure.
BMI: Body Mass Index.

The partial correlations between DBP and BMC in post-pubertal adolescents were not significant. Sub-division of the post-pubertal group based on gender revealed no significant correlations in girls (n=37); inverse correlations in boys (n=11) became stronger (r= -0.80, p=0.02). Sub-division of the pre-pubertal and pubertal group based on gender did not change the non-significant findings.

Table 3 shows partial correlations between anthropometric indices (weight, BMI, fat mass, lean mass), and BMC, SBP and DBP. Weight and lean mass were more strongly correlated with BMC and SBP as compared to BMI and fat mass. There were no significant correlations between anthropometric indices and DBP.

Hypertensive individuals were compared with normotensives using general linear models and results are presented in table 4.

Table 4. BMC MEANS OF HYPERTENSIVES VERSUS NORMOTENSIVES (ADJUSTED FOR BMI)

	BMC (g)
BOYS	
Hypertensives n=21	1437†
Normotensives n=84	1639
GIRLS	
Hypertensives n=25	1435†
Normotensives n=57	1620
PRE- AND PUBERTAL	
Hypertensives n=36	1323*
Normotensives n=103	1467
POST-PUBERTAL	
Hypertensives n=10	1776†
Normotensives n=38	2093

* significantly lower than normotensives ($p<0.005$).
† significantly lower than normotensives ($p<0.05$).
BMC: Bone Mineral Content.
BMI: Body Mass Index.

When BMI was adjusted for, hypertensive boys (n=21) had significantly lower BMC (1437 versus 1639 g; p=0.02) compared with normotensive boys (n=84); hypertensive girls (n=25) also had significantly lower BMC (1435 versus 1620 g; p=0.01) compared with normotensive girls (n=57). In the pre- and pubertal group, hypertensives (n=36) had significantly lower BMC (1323 versus 1467 g; p=0.004) compared with normotensives (n=103).

When this analysis was repeated in pre-pubertal children (Tanner stage 1-2) with the exclusion of pubertal (Tanner stage 3) children, results did not materially change; hypertensives (n=33) had significantly lower BMC (1309 versus 1444 g; p=0.009) compared with normotensives (n=90). Additionally, in the post-pubertal group, hypertensives (n=10) had significantly lower BMC (1776 versus 2093 g; p=0.01) compared with normotensives (n=38).

Conclusion

The results of this study suggest that there is a strong inverse association between systolic BP and BMC in adolescent boys. In addition, regardless of gender, hypertensives had significantly lower BMC compared with normotensives. There are several explanations for the inverse relationship between SBP and BMC and we believe that they include the complex interactions between blood pressure, insulin resistance, sex hormones, and bone mass.

In our previous study [14] of the metabolic profile of this sample, we found that there was a tendency for post-pubertal adolescents to have greater number of features of the metabolic syndrome than pre-pubertal and pubertal children; girls also tended to have a lower prevalence of features of the metabolic syndrome compared with boys. We previously [14] reported that insulin sensitivity is correlated negatively with SBP and DBP; insulin resistance may alter blood pressure by its effects on the sympathetic nervous system and by directly influencing renal sodium reabsorption [15]; high blood pressure may manifest due to lack of resistance to these secondary effects of insulin [16]. Other underlying mechanisms related to high BP and abnormalities in calcium metabolism which may ultimately influence peak bone mass include evidence of secondary increase in parathyroid gland activity [1,17], increase in urinary cyclic AMP [1,18], tendency to low serum ionized calcium [1,18-19], raised vitamin D levels [20], and increased intestinal calcium absorption [21].

Puberty is a critical time of flux and it raises a complex set of issues. The fact that we observed dramatic inverse correlations between SBP and BMC in post-pubertal boys but no such relationships in pre- and pubertal boys or in girls (table 2), may be explained by the profound rise in testosterone during puberty in boys and its atherogenic effects [22]. In adolescent boys, previous researchers have found a positive relationship between testosterone and SBP [23] and an inverse relationship between testosterone and HDL cholesterol [22]. Morrison et al. [22] conclude that changes in sex steroid hormones during puberty has significant effects on changes in lipid parameters with increasing testosterone having atherogenic effects and increasing estradiol having antiatherogenic effects. The fact that the relationship between SBP and BMC was not significant in post-pubertal girls (table 2) may also be explained by the antihypertensive [24], antiatherosclerotic [22,24], and osteogenic [25] properties of estrogen as well as the lack of the testosterone surge that is seen in boys. It is noteworthy that when we compared body size and composition in pre- versus post-pubertal boys (data not shown), we observed that although post-pubertal boys weighed more (81 kg versus 65 kg, p=0.006), they had significantly lower percent fat (29% versus 39%, p=0.000) than pre- and pubertal boys. These findings (from DXA) are consistent with those of Leccia et al. (from skinfold measurements) who observed reductions in percent body fat in 98 Italian pubertal boys [26]. Since obesity is known to increase estradiol in males by converting testosterone to estradiol and lowering testosterone [27], losing fat may have the opposite effect and may therefore be another plausible reason for why the adverse relationship between SBP and BMC is much more profound in post-pubertal boys. These tentative conclusions regarding the role of steroid hormones and their interaction with body composition, BP and BMC should be interpreted with caution until they are explored further in our future longitudinal investigations of this population and validated by other researchers.

This study, although the first to examine the relationship between BP and BMC in pediatrics, has a number of limitations that need to be addressed. First, this study was restricted to overweight Latino children of predominantly Mexican descent and is not necessarily generalizeable to children of other ethnic groups. Secondly, because body size is a powerful determinant of BMC [28] and BP [13], the fact that our population was overweight may also influence generalizeability of our findings. However, in order to rule out the confounders of the relationship between BP and BMC, all statistical analyses of this study adjusted for body weight and height or BMI. In addition, the cross-sectional nature of this study makes it difficult to prove causality. Nevertheless, we were able to appropriately and accurately test the specific hypotheses of the study. Further, the strength of the association (ie. correlation) between BMC and SBP in the entire cohort, although significant, was not strong ($r<0.30$). However, sub-group correlations based on puberty and gender were as high as 0.80. Moreover, results from the general linear models comparing BMC in hypertensive versus normotensive children complemented all correlations and were significantly lower in hypertensives in every single sub-group analysis. In addition, the strength of the correlations observed in the entire cohort are similar to those seen in adults of other studies; therefore, the physiological mechanisms explaining hypertensive bone loss in adults could perhaps also explain the inverse relationships observed in adolescents and would therefore enhance the biological plausibility of our findings.

In conclusion, SBP is inversely correlated with BMC in overweight adolescents; additionally, hypertensives have lower adjusted means of BMC than normotensives. These promising new findings suggest that hypertension may be a risk factor for osteopenia in overweight children and adolescents; this risk may be exacerbated in post-pubertal boys.

Acknowledgments

This work is a shorter version of a previous publication (*Am. J. Hypertens.* 2007; 20:190-196) and it has been presented in part at the 33rd European Symposium on Calcified Tissues, Prague, Czech Republic, May 10-14, 2006. This study was supported in part by grant R01 DK 59211 from the National Institutes of Health and by grant M01 RR 00043 from General Clinical Research Center, National Center for Research Resources awarded to the University of Southern California.

References

[1] McCarron DA, Pingree PA, Rubin RJ, Gaucher SM, Molitch M, Krutzik S: Enhanced parathyroid function in essential hypertension: a homeostatic response to a urinary calcium leak. *Hypertension* 1980;2:162-168.

[2] Matkovic V: Calcium and peak bone mass. *J. Intern Med.* 1992;231:151-160.

[3] Tsuda K, Nishio I, Masuyama Y: Bone mineral density in women with essential hypertension. *Am. J. Hypert.* 2001;14:704-707.

[4] Afghani A, Johnson CA: Resting blood pressure and bone mineral content are inversely related in overweight and obese Hispanic women. *Am. J. Hypert.* 2006;19:286-292.

[5] Perez-Castrillon JL, Justo I, Silva J, Sanz A, Igea R, Escudero P, Pueyo C, Diaz C, Hernandez G, Duenas A: Bone mass and bone modelling markers in hypertensive postmenopausal women. *J Hum Hypert* 2003;17:107-110.

[6] van Hooft IMS, Grobbee DE, Frolich M, Pols HAP, Hofman A: Alterations in calcium metabolism in young people at risk for primary hypertension. The Dutch Hypertension and Offspring Study. *Hypertension* 1993;21:267-272.

[7] Yamakawa H, Suzuki H, Nakamura M, Ohno Y, Saruta T: Disturbed calcium metabolism in offspring of hypertensive parents. *Hypertension* 1992;19:528-534.

[8] Cirillo M, Galletti F, Strazzullo P, Torielli L, Melloni MC: On the pathogenetic mechanism of hypercalciuria in genetically hypertensive rats of the Milan strain. *Am. J. Hypertens* 1989;2:741-746.

[9] Ogden CL, Flegal KM, Carroll MD, Johnson CL: Prevalence and Trends in Overweight Among U.S. Children and Adolescents, 1999-2000. *JAMA* 2002;288:1728-1732.

[10] Larijani B, Bekheirnia MR, Soltani A, Khalili-Far A, Adibi H, Jalili RB: Bone mineral density is related to blood pressure in men. *Am. J. Hum. Biol.* 2004; 16:168-171.

[11] American Diabetes Association: Type 2 diabetes in children and adolescents. Pediatrics 2000;105:671-680.

[12] National High Blood Pressure Education Program Working Group on Hypertension Control in Children and Adolescents: Update on the 1987 task force report on high blood pressure in children and adolescents: a working group report from the national high blood pressure education program. *Pediatrics* 1996;98:649-658.

[13] Rosner B, Prineas RJ, Loggie JM, Daniels SR: Blood pressure normograms for children and adolescents by height, sex, and age, in the United States. *J. Pediatr.* 1993;123:871-886.

[14] Cruz ML, Weigensberg MJ, Huang TTK, Ball G, Shaibi GQ, Goran MI: The metabolic syndrome in overweight Hispanic youth and the role of insulin sensitivity. *J. Clin. Endocrinol. Metab.* 2004;89:108-113.

[15] DeFronzo RA: The effect of insulin on renal sodium metabolism. A review with clinical implications. *Diabetologia* 1981;21:165-171.

[16] Anderson EA, Mark AL: The vasodilator action of insulin. Implications for the insulin hypothesis of hypertension. *Hypertension* 1993;21:136-141.

[17] Jorde R, Sundsfjord J, Haug E, Bonaa KH: Relation between low calcium intake, parathyroid hormone, and blood pressure. *Hypertension* 2000;35:1154-1159.

[18] Strazzullo P, Nunziata V, Cirillo M, Giannattasio R, Ferrara LA, Mattioli PL, Mancini M: Abnormalities of calcium metabolism in essential hypertension. *Clin. Sci.* 1983;65:137-141.

[19] McCarron DA: Low serum concentrations of ionized calcium in patients with hypertension. *N. Engl. J. Med.* 1982;307:226-228.

[20] Brickman AS, Nyby MD, von Hungen K, Eggena P, Tuck ML: Calcitropic hormones, platelet calcium, and blood pressure in essential hypertension. *Hypertension* 1990;16:515-522.

[21] Gadallah M, Massry SG, Bigazzi R, Horst RL, Eggena P, Campese VM: Intestinal absorption of calcium and calcium metabolism in patients with essential hypertension and normal renal function. *Am. J. Hypertens* 1991;4:404-409.

[22] Morrison JA, Barton BA, Biro FM, Sprecher DL: Sex hormones and the changes in adolescent male lipids: longitudinal studies in a biracial cohort. *J. Pediatr.* 2003;142:637-642.

[23] Shakov IUA, Riabinkina OIU, Maslennikov GIA, Isakova GL, Vorontsov VI: Sex hormones in dyslipoproteinemias and disorders of arterial blood pressure in boys 11-12 years of age. *Kardiologiia* 1989;29:81-86.

[24] Oparil S. Hormones and vasoprotection: *Hypertension 1*999;33:170-176.

[25] Armamento-Villereal R, Villereal DT, Avioli L, Civitelli R: Estrogen status and heredity are major determinants of pre-menopausal bone mass. *J. Clin. Invest.* 1992;90:2464-2471.

[26] Leccia G, Marotta T, Masella MR, Mottola G, Mitrano G, Golia F, Capitanata P, Guida L, Contaldo F, Ferrara LA: Sex-related influence of body size and sexual maturation on blood pressure in adolescents. *Eur. J. Clin. Nutr.* 1999;53:333-337.

[27] Zumoff B, Strain SW, Kream J, O'Connor J, Levin J, Fukushima DK: Obese young men have elevated estrogen levels, but obese premenopausal women do not. *Metabolism* 1981;30:1011-1014.

[28] Afghani A, Xie B, Wiswell RA, Gong J, Li Y, Johnson CA: Bone Mass of Asian adolescents in China: Influence of physical activity and smoking. *Med. Sci. Sports Exerc.* 2003;35:720-729.

In: Hypertension, Heredity and Stroke
Editor: Cristina Moratinos and Bruno Cardenas
ISBN 978-1-60741-496-4

Chapter 9

Hypertension and Obesity

Alfonso D. Torres [*] ***and Colette A. Gushurst***
Pediatric Nephrology, Pediatrics and Human Development Michigan State University/Kalamazoo Center for Medical Studies, Kalamazoo, Michigan, USA

Abstract

The link between obesity and hypertension is examined in this chapter. Underlying mechanisms include increase in sympathetic activity, sodium balance, renal tubular sodium reabsorption, glomerular filtration rate (GFR) and development of insulin resistance. The role of leptin is examined in the development of hypertension in obese adolescents. Also considered in this review are the definitions of hypertension and principles of management for obese youth with hypertension. Pharmacologic agents used for management of hypertension include diuretics, alpha blockers, beta blockers, angiotensin converting enzyme inhibitors (ACE inhibitors), angiotensin-2 receptor blockers (ARBs), and long acting calcium channel blockers. The importance of weight control, caloric restriction, and exercise in the management of obesity in youth is also stressed.

Introduction

World health organization (WHO) data indicates that one billion individual are overweight and over 300,000 obese. Epidemiologic data reveal that the prevalence rates of obesity are increasing not only in the industrialized nations but also in developing countries. The number of overweight and obese adults in the United States of America (USA) has dramatically increased in the last 20 years. Approximately 60 % of USA males and 51% of the USA females are overweight or obese [1]. Of particular concern is the relatively new phenomenon of increasing prevalence in overweigh and obesity in children and adolescents. This is an alarming problem observed in industrialized as well as developing countries and in the urban centers more than in the rural areas. Overweight was reported in 40.9% of Mexican-American adolescents (12-19 years of age) 40.9% while obesity was noted in 22.9%; males had a higher prevalence of overweight and obesity than females [2]. In Pavia, northern Italy, the percent of overweight and obese boys were 20.9% and 4% while percentages of overweight and obese girls were 14.7% and 1.1% respectively [3].

In Pune, India the prevalence of overweight base on BMI was 27.5% in boys and 20.9 % in girls; hypertension was present in 12% of the overweight boys and in 9.75% of girls while the prevalence of hypertension increased with the increase in BMI [4]. In Lausanne Switzerland, of 2507 children studied with a mean standard deviation (SD) age 12.3 (0.5) years, 2.2 % were found to be hypertensive; of the hypertensive children, 16.1% of the boys and 12.4% of the girls were overweight or obese based on the CDC criteria of BMI > 85th percentile [5]. In a study in Poland (city of Lodz), involving 25,309 children and adolescents between 7-18 years of age, the mean prevalence of overweight was 15.1%; 13.2% of the girls and 17% of the boys were found to be overweight.6 Obesity was found in 4.4% of the boys and in 2.9 % of the girls [6]. Prehypertension was found in 11.1% and hypertension in 4.9 %; hypertension was more prevalent in the younger group ages 7-13 years than in the older group's age 14-19 years [6].

Similar observations have been made in Germany, China, and other countries. In the United States the prevalence of obesity increased from 5% to 13% in boys and from 5% to 9% in girls between 1996-1970 and 1988-1991 respectively [7]. In the United States, disparity exists in childhood and adolescent prevalence of obesity between regions and states of the Country [7]. South and central regions of the United States have an obesity prevalence of 18% while the mountain region has the lowest prevalence of 11.4% [7]. Children in West Virginia, Kentucky, Tennessee, Texas, and North Carolina all have an adjusted obesity prevalence >18.3%; this is over twice the odds of been obese than their Utah counterparts who have an adjusted prevalence of 10.4% [7]. Socioeconomic status, neighborhood, social capital, television viewing, recreational computer use, and physical activities account for 55% of the regional and states differences in the prevalence of obesity [7].

Substantial differences exist in the prevalence of overweight and obesity among different ethnic groups. African-American women and Mexican-American of both sexes have the highest prevalence of overweight in the United States today. However, the "epidemic" proportions of overweight and obesity can not be explained on the basis of familial or genetic factors alone. As a consequence of technologic advances over the past 30 years in agriculture, industry, communications, transport, commerce and medicine have brought changes in lifestyle all over the world, promoting a sedentary, self gratifying lifestyle in large number of children and adolescents. Education about appropriated nutrition and the importance of participation in physical activities has lagged behind [8].

Overweight and obesity are not variations of normal growth of children and adolescents, but that of illnesses requiring intervention. Excessive weight gain is an important risk for

* Correspondence: Alfonso D Torres, MD, Pediatric Nephrology Director, Michigan State University/Kalamazoo Center for Medical Studies, 1000 Oakland Drive, Kalamazoo, MI 49008-1284 United States. Tel: 269-337-6450; Fax: 269-337-6474; E-mail: Torres@kcms.msu.edu

comorbidities involving multiple organ systems: endocrine, cardiovascular, gastrointestinal, pulmonary, orthopedic, neurologic, dermatologic, and psychosocial. Clinical manifestations of overweight and obesity are many, including those listed in table 1.

Table 1. Complications of obesity

Hypertension
Type 2 Diabetes
Cardiovascular diseases
Cerebrovascular diseases
Sleep apnea
Back pain
Osteoarthritis
Non-alcohol-related fatty liver infiltration
Kidney diseases
Malignancies
Psychosocial disturbances

Based on the current prevalence of adolescent obesity in the United States, the prevalence of obesity in 35-years-olds will be in the range of 30% to 37% in men and 34% to 44% in women by the year 2020. A total increase in the number of patients with cardiovascular diseases is also expected to occur. Deaths secondary to coronary heart disease will increase in number and will occur in younger individuals as they approach middle age [9]. Recently a meta-analysis epidemiologic study involving 247 published papers indicated that there was a strong positive association between BMI and risk for kidney disease outcomes [10]. The authors concluded that 24.2% and 33.9% of kidney diseases among American men and women respectably (versus 13.8% in men and 24.9% in women in other industrialized countries) could be related to overweight and obesity [10]. Obesity by itself is clearly linked to glomerulomegaly and to a secondary form of focal segmental glomerulosclerosis, likely on the bassis of a hyperfiltration mechanism [11].

Obesity and Hypertension

The relationship between obesity and hypertension is well documented in children and adolescents, with blood pressure following an almost linear correlation though time; hypertension develops more often in those individuals that have been obese for over five years. Obesity is clearly related to type-2 diabetes mellitus and systemic arterial hypertension. Type 2 diabetes mellitus and hypertension are major risk complications of the development of coronary heart disease and chronic renal disease. Abundant clinical observations indicated that hypertension improves with reduction of body weight. Animal experimental observations that are highly reproducible demonstrate predictable elevation in blood pressure in association with high fat diets in dogs and rabbits as well as obese human beings [12].

How Obesity Induces Hypertension?

Experimental data in obese animals and clinical observations in obese humans are associated with hemodynamic, neurohumoral, and renal changes that include increased arterial pressure, heart rate, and cardiac output. There is increase in sympathetic activity, sodium balance, renal tubular sodium reabsorption, glomerular filtration rate (GFR), and development of insulin resistance [13]. Endothelial dysfunction and carotid intimal thickening are also observed in children and adolescents with obesity and hypertension.

The increase in cardiac output observed in obese individuals is not necessarily directed to the increased adipose tissue. The change in blood flow is more likely due to general vasodilation induced by increase metabolic rate in many organs given the increase in organ size; this vasodilation is probably mediated by nitrous oxide (NO) produced by the endothelium and seems to occur early, before the development of vascular disease.

Increase heart rate early in obesity seems to be mediated by diminution of the parasympathetic tone in the heart, rather than change in sympathetic activity [14]. There are many studies however, linking obesity with hypertension and the role of the sympathetic nervous system activity in this relationship [15]. Ethnicity may be an important factor to consider given the fact that sympathetic nervous system activity as well as propensity to obesity and hypertension differ with different ethnic groups. In obesity, sympathetic nerve system activity is increased in skeletal muscle, as detected by microneurography that measures muscle sympathetic nerve activity; this technique has shown consistent elevation of such nerve activity in obesity [16]. One detrimental effect is to increase sympathetic activity to the peripheral vasculature resulting in vasoconstriction with time. Pharmacologic inhibition of the sympathetic nervous system(SNS) with alpha and beta blockers reduces blood pressure to a greater extent in obese than in lean individuals.

Examination of norepinephrine spillover in obesity has shown regional hyperactivity in the kidneys. Increase SNS activity in the kidneys cav lead to sodium retention and abnormal hemodynamics resulting in increased blood pressure. Patients with obesity-associated hypertension present with positive sodium balance and expanded extracellular volume. In normal subjects, expanded extracellular volume triggers mild increase in blood pressure, resulting in a significant sodium excretion by the kidney and restoration of normal volume. This phenomenon is known as "pressure natriuresis" and functions as a physiologic back-up system for preservation of the extracellular volume. In hypertensive obese individuals, pressure natriuresis is impaired, requiring higher blood pressure to excrete a sodium load. In experimental obese animals, sympathetic renal denervation attenuates renal sodium retention associated with high fat diet. Several other potential mechanism have been implicated in the activation of the SNS in obesity associated hypertension, including hyperinsulinemia, increase levels of free fatty acids, impaired baroreceptor reflexes, obstructive sleep apnea, and cytokines release from adipocytes. Visceral obesity is a high risk for obstructive sleep apnea that is often seen in association with hypertension. These patients have an increased peripheral chemoreflex response to hypoxia resulting in activation of the SNS.

There is also a clear link between visceral fat accumulation and SNS activity and hypertension is mediated through the visceral fat production of leptin. Leptin is a protein produced mainly by visceral adipose tissue that acts in the central nervous system. Leptin plasma concentration is elevated in obese humans [17]. One of the leptin pathways in the hypothalamus involves stimulation of the pro-opiomelacortin neurons in the arcuate nucleus that then send projections to the paraventricular nucleus and lateral hypothalamus releasing a-melanocyte-stimulating hormone (a-MSH) which is an agonist for acting on melanocortin receptors 3/4 (MC3/4-R). These neurons projections act on the nucleus of the solitary tract in the midbrain affecting changes in appetite, SNS activity, and blood pressure [18]. Currently leptin secreted by adipocytes is the main factor linking obesity with increased sympathetic nerve system activity and hypertension [19].

It is well known that the kidney contains all the elements for intrinsic activation of the renin-angiotensin-aldosterone system (RAAS). The intrarenal RAAS seems to be involved in hypertension associated with visceral obesity despite the fact that there is sodium retention and expansion of the extracellular volume. Possible explanations for the activation of renin secretion may involve activation of the sympathetic renal nerves and decrease sodium delivery to the macula densa due to increase sodium reabsorption early in the proximal tubule and the loop of Henle. In addition, increased renal pressure induced by visceral and intrarenal fat can stimulate renin secretion as seen in the peg kidney. Increase activity of RAAS causes efferent arteriole vasoconstriction and may result in hyperfiltration and nephrosclerosis. Aldosterone has direct mineralocorticoid receptor agonist effects resulting in increased sodium reabsorption in the cortical collecting duct and increasing blood pressure. Additionally, aldosterone is considered to promote fibrosis in organs such as the heart. Mineralocorticoid blockers are useful in the management of obese hypertensive patients.

The view that overweight and obesity represent simply a mater of caloric deposits is obsolete; we are learning that the adipose tissue is a very complex biologic system with surprising number of functions interacting with other organ systems including those listed in table 2. Adipose tissues are the source of numerous hormones, cytokines, growth factors, and complement factors that promote inflammation. Endothelial dysfunction eventually leads to promotion of vascular wall stiffness and is correlated with increase in carotid intimal-medial wall thickness [20].

Table 2. Interactions of adipose tissue

Central and Peripheral Nervous systems
Endocrine system
Cardiovascular system
Musculoskeletal system
Renal system
Immune system

A recently published epidemiologic meta-analysis involving 247 published papers from 1980 to 2006 demonstrated that compared with normal individuals, overweight and obese persons had significantly higher risk for kidney disease.21 The pooled relative risks (RRS) were 1.4 (1.30-1.50) for overweight and 1.83 (1.78-2.17) for obesity [21]. The association between obesity and kidney disease was stronger in women with RR=1.92 (1.78-2.07) than in men with RR=1.49 (1.36-1.63) [21]. This study indicated that there is a positive association between BMI and risk for kidney disease outcomes. The authors concluded that 24.2% and 33.9% of kidney diseases among men and women respectively in the United States versus 13.8% in men and 24.9% in women in other industrialized countries could be related to overweight and obesity [10].

Definitions of Hypertension in Children and Adolescents

The Fourth Report on the diagnosis, evaluation, and treatment of high blood pressure in children and adolescents uses blood pressure percentiles based upon demographic data from the National Health and Nutritional Examination Surveys (NHANES), taking in consideration information on gender, age, height, and blood pressure measurements on three separated occasions [21].

Table 3 lists hypertension definitions. Both systolic and diastolic blood pressures are of equal importance and the higher value determines the severity of the hypertension. The blood pressure should be measured in at least three different occasions to establish the diagnosis of hypertension. Stage 1 hypertension (see table 3) allows more time for evaluation. Treatment may be initiated with no pharmacologic approach that includes lifestyle modification such a weight loss, diet, and exercise. Stage-2 hypertension (se table 3) is more likely to be secondary hypertension and requires more rapid evaluation as well as initiation of pharmacologic intervention.

Table 3. Definitions of hypertension

1. Normal - systolic and diastolic blood pressure < 90 percentile
2. Prehypertension – Systolic and/or diastolic blood pressure >90th percentile but < 95th percentile, or if BP exceeds 120/80 mmHg even if <90th percentile
3. Stage 1 Hypertension – Systolic and/or diastolic BP between the 95th percentile and 5 mmHg above the 99th percentile.
4. Stage 2 Hypertension – Systolic and/or diastolic BP > 99% percentile + 5mmHg.

Treatment of Hypertension in Obese Adolescents

The treatment of the hypertensive obese adolescent is based on the same principles of treatment as used for management of other causes of hypertension. It is important to obtain a comprehensive history including a family history. The physical examination should be aimed to find possible secondary causes of hypertension that can be amenable to specific therapy, resulting in the cure or amelioration of the hypertension. Appropriate laboratory studies (see table 4) are helpful in investigating secondary forms of hypertension. Secondary forms of hypertension are more common in preadolescent children. Essential hypertension is more often seen in families with positive histories for hypertension and obesity.

Table 4. Selective list of key laboratory tests in hypertension evaluation

Urinalysis
Creatinine
Urea nitrogen
Electrolytes
Others

The cornerstone of management of hypertension secondary to obesity is body weight reduction and limiting caloric intake is necessary. Behavior modification is also very important. Better results are obtained by caloric restriction, behavior changes, and regular exercise [22]. The experience for weight reduction with pharmacologic agents is limited and in general not recommended in the United States for adolescents. There are reports of a few small series of morbidly obese adolescents with BMI > 40 Kg/ M^2 that have treated surgically for weight reduction [23]. However, lifestyle modification with behavior changes and exercise continues to be the best management option for most patients, particularly prehypertensive and stage 1 hypertensive adolescents. Adolescents with stage 1 hypertension should be monitored every few months. If the hypertension becomes more severe or symptomatic, stage 2 hypertension is diagnosed, and pharmacologic treatment is indicated.

Pharmacologic Therapy for Obese Hypertensive Adolescents

Several classes of medication are able to successfully control elevated blood pressure in adolescents as listed in table 5. The decision to utilize a specific medication however, requires consideration of the potential undesirable side effects, including metabolic consequences. It is well known that diuretics decrease blood pressure and offer cardiovascular protection in many hypertensive patients and are recommended as the fist line therapy for hypertensive adults. However in obese patients, there is an increase in the fasting blood glucose (FBG) levels in patients that were started on treatment with thiazides for hypertension. The magnitude of change in FBG and the development of new onset diabetes mellitus after thiazide initiation have been associated with increase in BMI and base line FBG [24]. Additionally, diuretic use is associated with electrolyte disturbances, particularly hypokalemia, hyponatremia, and abnormalities in uric acid metabolism.

Table 5. Medications for treatment of hypertension in adolescents

Diuretics
Alpha blockers
Beta blockers
Angiotensin converting enzyme inhibitors (ACE inhibitors)
Angiotensin-2 receptor blockers (ARBs)
Long acting calcium channel blockers

The experience with beta blockers for the treatment of hypertension in pediatrics is extensive. In the older adult population, beta blockers are particularly beneficial after myocardial infarction. However, beta blockers make glucose control more difficult; they are also associated with increased lipid levels and make it more difficult for the individual to loss weight. In younger obese individuals, other metabolically more neutral alternatives for treatment of hypertension are available.

Increasing experience in the use of angiotensin converting enzyme (ACE) inhibitors and angiotensin-2 receptor blockers (ARBs) is accumulating in the treatment of hypertensive adolescents and in children. In general, these medications are well tolerated by adolescents. Precautions are necessary in those adolescents with decrease renal function because for the risk of aggravating the decreased glomerular filtration rate and the development of hyperkalemia. These drugs are effective in controlling the elevated blood pressure, and because most are long acting medications, compliance is better. One drawback with these medications is the possibility of development of angioedema, a rare but serious complication. Another important consideration is their use in the adolescent female at risk of becoming pregnant given the teratogenic effects of ACEs and ARBs in the fetus.

Long acting calcium channel blockers are used for different forms of hypertension and are well tolerated in adolescents. They are associated with less metabolic abnormalities than diuretic or beta blockers [25]. The dihydropyridine calcium channel blocker, amlodipine, induces tachycardia and ankle edema that are of no clinic consequence; gum hypertrophy is also noted. Recent publications seem to indicate that that long term thiazide diuretics can increase fasting blood glucose and BMI levels and predispose to development of diabetes mellitus in hypertensive patients [24,25]. These studies indicate that the selection of antihypertensive medications is important to prevent or diminish the undesirables metabolic consequences that may be induced in susceptible individuals by certain medications.

Conclusions

Overweight and obesity in adolescents is now a global problem affecting developed and developing societies around the world. It is predictable that childhood and adolescent obesity will translate into adulthood obesity and its consequent morbidities including hypertension, hyperlipidemia, as well as type 2 diabetes mellitus and cardiovascular diseases. The causes of overweight and obesity in children and adolescents are the result of excessive caloric intake and concomitant decline in levels of physical activity in association with various socioeconomic, cultural, and genetic factors. There are populations that are at higher risk than others to be affected by these factors, including Asian Pacific Islanders, Australian Aborigine, African American Hispanics, and Native Americans; however no populations are exempt.

Adolescent hypertension is one of the co-morbidities of obesity that can be detected, prevented, and treated. The diagnosis of hypertension in adolescents in the United States is based on the recently published guidelines [21]. The cornerstone in the treatment of obesity-associated hypertension in adolescents is weight reduction by decreased caloric intake, behavior modification, and exercise. Organized physical activities and sport programs at schools and/or in the community in important in this regard. When pharmacologic therapy becomes necessary the prescribing physician needs to become familiar with the different antihypertensive medications as well as their side effects noted in obese diabetic patients, in those with cardiovascular diseases, and in patients with diminished kidney function. The best approach to the management of the obese "epidemic" is prevention and in this regard, health education of the population at large is critical.

References

[1] Jensen MD. Obesity. In: Goldman L, Ausiello D, eds. Cecil medicine, 23rd ed. Philadelphia, PA: Saunders Elsevier, 2008:1643-52.

[2] Forrest KY, Leeds MJ. Prevalence and associated factors of overweight among Mexican-American adolescents. *J. Am. Diet Assoc.* 2007;107(10):797-800.

[3] Turconi G, Guarcello M, Maccarini L, Bazzano R, Zacardo A, Roggi C. BMI values and other anthropometric and functional measurements as predictors of obesity in selected group of adolescents. *Eur. J. Nutr.* 2006;45(3):136-43.

[4] Rao S, Kanade A, Kelkar R. Blood Pressure among overweight adolescents from urban school children in Pune, India. *Eur. J. Clin. Nutr.*, 2007;61(5):633-41.

[5] Chiolero A, Cachat F, Burnier M, Paccaud F, Bovet P. Prevalence of hypertension in schoolchildren based in repeated measurements and association with overweight. *J. Hypertension* 2007;25(11):2209-17.

[6] Ostroswska-Nawarycz L, Nawaricz T. Prevalence of excessive body weight and high blood pressure in children and adolescents in the city of Lodz. *Kardiol. Pol.* 2007;65(9):1079- 87.

[7] Singh GK. Kogan MD, VanDick PC. Multilevel analysis of state and regional disparities of children and adolescents obesity in the United States. *J. Community Health* 2007;34:222-5.

[8] Pazmino P A, Pazmino A K, Diabetic renal failure in Texas: Influence of ethnicity and household income. *Tex. Med.* 2003;99:57-65.

[9] Bibbins-Domingo K, Coxon P, Pletcher MJ, Lightwood J, Goldman L. Adolescent overweight and future adult coronary heart disease. *N. Engl. J. Med.* 2007;357:2371-9.

[10] Wang Y, Chen X, Song Y, Caballero B, Cheskin LJ. Association between obesity and kidney disease: A systemic review and meta-analysis: *Kidney Int.* 2008;73:19-33.

[11] Kambham N, Markowitz GS, Valeri AM, et al. Obesity and related glomerulopathy: An emerging epidemic. *Kidney Int.* 2001;59:1498-1509.

[12] Hall JE Brands MW, Dixon WN, et al Obesity induced-hypertension: Renal function and systemic hemodynamics. *Hypertension* 1993;22:292-9.

[13] Messereli FH, Christie B, DeCarvalho JG, Obesity and essential hypertension: Hemodynamics, intravascular volume, sodium excretion, and plasma renain activity. *Arch. Intern. Med.* 1981; 141:81-5.

[14] Vaz M, Jennings G, Turner A, et al. Regional sympathetic nervous activity and oxygen consumption in obese normotensive human subjects: *Circulation* 1997;96:3423-9.

[15] Lambert E, Staznicky M, Esler M, Dawood T, Hotchkin E, Lambert G. Differing patterns of sympathoexitation in normal-weight and obesity related hypertension. *Hypertension* 2007;50(50):862-8.

[16] Corry DB, Tuck ML. Obesity, hypertension and sympathetic nerve system activity. Curr *Hypertens Rep.* 1999;1(2):119-26.

[17] Haynes WG, Interaction between leptin and sympathetic system activity in hypertension. *Curr. Hypertens Rep.* 2000;2(3):311-8.

[18] John E. Hall, Alexander A da Silva, Elizabeth Brandon, et al. Pathophysiology of obesity induced hypertension and target organ damage. In: Lip GYH, Hall JE, eds. Comprehensive hypertension. Philadelphia, PA: Mosby Elsevier, 2007:441-68.

[19] Francischetti EA, Genelhu VA. Obesity-hypertension: An ongoing pandemic. *Int. J. Clin. Pract.* 2007;61(2):269-80.

[20] Sorof JM, Turner J, Martin DS, et al. Cardiovascular risks factors and sequelae in hypertensive children identified by referral versus school base screening. *Hypertension* 2004;43:214-8.

[21] The Fourth Report on diagnosis, evaluation and treatment of high blood pressure in children and adolescents. Bethesda, MD: Nat Heart Lung Blood Inst Health. *Pediatrics* 2004;114:555-76.

[22] Rocchini AP, Cutch V, Anderson J, Becker D, Martin M, Mark C. Blood pressure in obese adolescents, effect of weight loss. *Pediatrics* 1998;82(1):16-23.

[23] Widhalm K, Dietrich S, Prager G, Silberhummer G, et al. Bariatric surgery in morbidly obese adolescents: A 4-year follow-up of ten patients. *Int. J. Pediatr. Obes.* 2008;3(suppl 1):78-82.

[24] Siegel D, Meier J, Maas C, Lopez J. Swislocki AL. The effect of body mass index on fasting blood glucose after initiation of thiazide therapy in hypertensive patients. *Am. J. Hypertension.* 2008; [Epub ahead of print]

[25] Gupta AK, Dahlof B, Dobson j, Sever PS, Wedel H, Poulter NR; on behalf of ASCOT Investigators. Determinants of new-onset diabetes Among 19,251 hypertensive patients randomized in the ASCOT-BPLA Trial and relative influence of antihypertensive medication. *Diabetes Care* 2008; [Epub ahead of print].

In: Hypertension, Heredity and Stroke
Editor: Cristina Moratinos and Bruno Cardenas

ISBN 978-1-60741-496-4

Chapter 10

Arterial Hypertension in Children after the Surgical Repair of Aortic Coarctation

Tomasz Florianczyk, Bozena Werner, Jacek Skiendzielewski and Piotr Wieniawski
Department of Pediatric Cardiology and General Pediatrics.
The Medical University of Warsaw

Abstract

Arterial hypertension is one of main clinical symptoms of aortic coarctation in children and could be also observed after the surgical treatment despite of good result of the surgery.

The prevalence of arterial hypertension in children successfully treated due to coarctation of the aorta ranges from 7% to 75% according to various authors. The risk of arterial hypertension rises with the patient's age and follow-up period after surgery. Moreover the incidence of postcoarctectomy hypertension is quite low in children operated in infancy in comparison to these who undergo surgical treatment in older age.

Arterial hypertension could be observed immediately after the surgical treatment as a result of sympathetic nervous system hyperstymulation due to baroreceptor reflex or increased activity of the complex of rennin-angiotensin–aldosteron. We observed a hypertension crisis in infant just after the balloon angioplasty of aortic recoarctation who underwent the procedure 4 months after the primary surgical treatment.

In etiology of late postcoarctectomy hypertension the following factors are considered: residual aortic coarctation, decreased sensitivity of baroreceptor reflex, increased activity of the rennin-angiotensin-aldosteron complex and rise of vasopressin secretion.

In evaluated group of 93 patients after the successful surgical repair of aortic coarctation hypertension was found in 24,7% of cases based on sphygmomanometer measurement and in 19,3% of cases using ABPM. In children operated in infancy the prevalence was 11,4 %, while in those operated in older age 34,4%.

Introduction

Coarctation of the aorta (CoA) involves stenosis of the main artery in the anatomical isthmus located just distal to the origin of the left subclavian artery. This accounts for 5-8% of all congenital heart and great vessel diseases [1-4]. Arterial hypertension is a typical symptom in this condition. Three pathomechanisms are presumed to underlie hypertension: increased vascular resistance associated with the coarctation, impaired baroreflex due to constant stimulation of aortic arch baroreceptors by elevated arterial blood pressure as well as increased activity of the renin-angiotensin-aldosterone system caused by decreased in renal perfusion secondary to low blood pressure distally to the aortic isthmus [5]. Despite good outcomes of surgical treatment, increased incidence of hypertension is also observed in patients after surgical repair of coarctation of the aorta. The cause of this relationship remains unknown; however; it has been recently highlighted that hypertension following CoA repair is only a dominant manifestation of systemic vascular disease involving fragmentation of the elastic fibers, enhanced fibrosis and presence of necrotic foci within the media of the ascending and descending aortic wall [6-8]. The theory of systemic vascular changes in the CoA is supported by an increased risk of intracranial aneurysms [9].

Study Aim

The aim of this study was to assess the incidence of arterial hypertension in children with successfully repaired coarctation of the aorta with respect to their age at the time of cardiosurgery.

Study Population and Design

The analysis was performed in 93 children, including 60 boys and 33 girls aged from 2 days to 19.16 years old (mean 12.90 ± 6.22 years) with successful outcome of the CoA surgical repair. The successful result of surgical repair refers to normal blood flow profile through the aortic isthmus in conventional Doppler Imaging and systolic pressure gradient between the upper and lower limbs below 20 mm Hg using manometer and Doppler measurements. Patient age at the time of repair was form 2 days to 13.52 years (mean 1.83 ± 3.01 years). Sixty one children (65.6%) were operated on within their first 12 months of life (30 in the neonatal period and 31 at the age from 2 to 12 months), while 32 children (34.4%) underwent cardiosurgery above their first year of age. The average follow-up period was 8.57 ± 3.72 years.

The control group comprised 34 healthy children, including 22 boys and 12 girls aged from 6.05 to 18.02 years (mean 12.08 ± 3.03 years).

All children had standard blood pressure measurement using a sphygmomanometer and an ambulatory blood pressure monitoring (ABPM).

Standard blood pressure measurements were carried out with the use of Riester mercury manometer according to measurement principles and normal blood pressure levels tables in children provided in the Fourth Report on the Diagnosis, Evaluation, and Treatment of High Blood Pressure in Children and Adolescents [10]. Normal blood pressure was diagnosed if systolic and diastolic blood pressure did not exceed the 90th percentile matched to the sex, age and height. Prehypertension was confirmed in children with systolic or diastolic blood pressure from ≥ 90th percentile to < 95th percentile with respect to sex, age and height or above 120/80 mm Hg. Arterial hypertension was diagnosed in patients with systolic and diastolic blood pressure ≥ 95th percentile based on sex, age, and height. Children with normal diastolic blood pressure and with systolic blood pressure of ≥ 90th percentile or ≥ 95th percentile were diagnosed as having systolic prehypertension or systolic hypertension, respectively. Hypertension rate was analyzed in the whole study group as well as in the subgroups of 61 children operated on below the age of 1 year and 32 children operated on at higher age.

ABPM cuff was placed on the right arm and SpaceLabs oscillometric device with ABP Report Management System were used for recording and analysis. The measurements were performed in 15-minute intervals in the awakeness period from 08:00 to 20:00 and every 30 minutes during sleep from 0:00 to 6:00. Mean 24-hour systolic and diastolic blood pressures were evaluated in relation to ABPM reference ranges matched to sex and height. ABPM normal ranges by Borowski et al. [11 were applied in children taller than 140 cm, whereas Soergel et al. [12] normal ranges were used for shorter ones. Arterial hypertension was diagnosed based on ABPM if mean 24-hour systolic and diastolic blood pressure levels were above the 95th percentile for sex and height, while systolic hypertension was diagnosed in subjects with mean 24-hour systolic blood pressure levels above the 95th percentile and with normal diastolic pressure.

The comparative analysis of mean systolic and diastolic blood pressure from standard measurement and mean 24-hour levels from ABPM in children from the study and control groups were performed with t-Student test for independent variables. Chi-square test with Yates' correction was applied for the analysis of arterial hypertension rates.

Results

Mean values of systolic and diastolic blood pressure from the standard measurements and mean 24-hour systolic and diastolic blood pressures from ABPM in children after surgical repair of coarctation of the aorta and in the controls are presented in Table 1. Systolic hypertension was diagnosed in 23 (24.7%) of 93 patients in the study group and systolic prehypertension was confirmed in 4 children (4.4%). The other 66 children (70.9%) from the study group were normotensive. Systolic hypertension rate in the study population was significantly higher in comparison to controls ($p<0.01$). No significant differences were found ($p>0.05$) with respect to systolic prehypertension between the study and control groups.

Out of 61 children operated within their first 12 months of age, 7 (11.4%) were found to have systolic hypertension while 11 hypertensive ones (34.4%) were in the group operated at later age. The incidence of hypertension in the children with repair performed above the age of 12 months was significantly higher than in children operated on as infants or neonates (p<0.01).

Table 1. Results of blood pressure measurements using standard mercury sphygmomanometer and ABPM in children from the study and control group

	SBP /mmHg/	DBP /mmHg/	ABPM-SBP /mmHg/	ABPM-DBP /mmHg/
Study group	116,38 ± 11,23	60,61 ± 6,39	124,56 ± 7,42	67,09 ± 6,03
Control group	103,67 ± 10,59	58,91 ± 6,52	114,29 ± 8,98	65,56 ± 4,72
p	<0,01	NS	<0,001	NS

SBP– Systolic blood pressure in standard mercury sphygmomanometer measurement.
DBP – Diastolic blood pressure in standard mercury sphygmomanometer measurement.
ABPM-SBP – 24-hours systolic blood pressure in ABPM.
ABPM-DBP –24-hours diastolic blood pressure in ABPM.

Based on ABPM, high blood pressure was found in 18 children (19.3%) from the study group, including 17 (18.2%) ones in whom systolic hypertension was confirmed and one diagnosed with arterial hypertension (1.1%). The incidence of arterial hypertension and isolated systolic hypertension was significantly higher as compared to the control group (p<0.01).

In the ABPM 15 of 23 subjects with elevated systolic blood pressure in the standard measurement were not established to have arterial hypertension although in another 8 systolic hypertension was confirmed. Moreover, 8 normotensive children and 2 prehypertensive ones in the standard measurement had hypertension based on ABPM.

Discussion

Late hypertension is an important clinical problem in children after surgical repair of coarctation of the aorta despite continued improvement of surgical technique and possibility to perform the surgical treatment in the neonatal and early infantile periods.

Arterial hypertension in patients after repair of CoA may be observed just after the cardiosurgery as an early or late paradoxical hypertension, and late in the postoperative period as late hypertension. Moreover, high blood pressure in this patient population occurs in cases of postsurgical re-coarctation.

Early hypertension occurs within 12-24 hours after the cardiosurgery for aortic coarctation and is associated with increased sympathetic tone secondary to baroreceptor activation in the aortic arch and carotid bodies. Late paradoxical hypertension is most frequently observed in 2-5 days after the cardiosurgery. It results from increased activation of renin-angiotensin-aldosterone system. It should be noted that in both, early and late paradoxical hypertension, the blood pressure values may be even higher than in the preoperative period. Paradoxical hypertension may also occur after balloon angioplasty of re-coarctation as it was seen in an 4-month-old infant treated at our center [13].

Late hypertension in patients with successful results of aortic coarctation repair may occur immediately or later after the cardiosurgery, following the normotensive period. The cause of high blood pressure in patients after surgical repair of CoA remains unknown.

In our study the incidence of arterial hypertension based on standard measurement in children after surgical repair of CoA was 24.70% and was statistically significantly higher as compared to the healthy group. The available literature reports the late arterial hypertension after CoA repair in 7% to 75% of patients [14-17]. Hypertension diagnosed based on ABPM was found in 19.3% of the study children, including 18.2% of children with systolic hypertension, and 1.1% of children with both, systolic and diastolic hypertension. ABPM allowed for exclusion of arterial hypertension in 15 children with high blood pressure diagnosed with the standard measurements. It may be associated with white-coat hypertension which occurs in 27% to 79% of in children and adolescents [18,19]. In the analysis of our 212 ABPM records, performed form 2005 to 2007 in children suspected of hypertension, a white-coat hypertension was confirmed in 32.6% of patients [20].

We believe that ABPM should be performed in all children after CoA repair in order to confirm or exclude hypertension, regardless of results of standard blood pressure measurement.

In 8 studied children found to be normotensive on standard blood pressure measurement, ABPM revealed hypertension which may result from exercise-induced hypertensive response. Exercise induces hypertension in patients with normal blood pressure in the standard measurement and normotensive in the ABPM should be an indication for exercise stress test.

The incidence of hypertension based on the standard blood pressure measurements in children operated on at the age of above 12 months was 34.4% and was higher compared with the children treated in the neonatal or infantile periods, where it equaled 11.4%. It has been highlighted that the incidence of hypertension in this patient population increases with the age at the time of cardiosurgery being lower in children operated on before 12 months of age and ranging form 7% to 21% [15,17,19,21-24]. The repair of CoA at the later age is associated with increased mortality which ranges from 7.5% to 18% and is related to cardiovascular disorders such as coronary artery disease, hemorrhagic stroke and rupture of aortic aneurysms [21,25].

The average postoperative follow-up in children from the study group was 8.57±3.72 years. Vriend et al. [26] reported that the incidence of hypertension in patients after repair of CoA increased along with the duration of postoperative period; the meta-analysis of published data showed the rate reaching 20% to 40% within 10–20 years after the cardiosurgery.

Patients after repair of the CoA present mainly with systolic hypertension which may stand for the thesis that hypertension results in this patient population from enhanced rigidity and decreased compliance of the systemic arteries proximal to the coarctation. This hypothesis was confirmed by a number of clinical studies [16,27,28]. Brili et al. [29] showed that increased systemic stiffness proximal to the coarctation of the aorta may also follow chronic inflammatory reaction of the vascular walls which was observed during pre- and post-repair periods. Sehested et al. [30] showed elevated collagen levels and reduced number of myocytes in the arterial walls proximal to the coarctation.

The cause of late arterial hypertension in patients with surgical CoA repair has not been established so far. Except for the increased aortic stiffness, also number of other pro-hypertensive factors was considered for this group of patients such as increased activity of renin-angiotensin-aldosterone system, baroreflex impairment, disturbance of the autonomic control of vascular resistance, presence of residual postoperative stenosis at the isthmus or disturbed aortic arch geometry [6,31-38].

The importance of impaired reactivity of the great arteries in induction of high blood pressures in patients after CoA repair has been currently highlighted which may be associated with endothelial and muscular layer dysfunction [37]. Gardiner et al. [39] showed decreased brachial artery reactivity with maintained normal relaxation response in the radial artery in patients with previous repair of CoA which confirms impaired reactivity of the great arteries proximally to the aortic isthmus in this group of patients. Those authors also documented that the reactivity decrease correlated with the age the time of cardiosurgery and was independent of the patient's age and body mass index. It is still controversial if reactivity disturbances are the cause or consequence of the arterial hypertension. Initially it was believed that endothelial function disturbances resulted from arterial hypertension [40,41]. However, the recent reports show predominant role of decreased vascular reactivity in hypertensive patients [42].

The improvement of care and treatment effects in children and adolescents with late arterial hypertension after surgical repair of coarctation of the aorta require further studies on hypertensive disease etiology in this population.

Conclusion

1. All children after surgical repair of the coarctation of the aorta require regular monitoring of blood pressure using standard measurements and ABPM.
2. Children with good outcomes of surgical repair of the coarctation of the aorta often develop hypertension in the long-term follow-up.
3. Systolic hypertension is the most common clinical problem in children after surgical repair of the coarctation of the aorta.

References

[1] Cheng Ch., Wu M., Wang J.: Ductus-dependent aortic coarctation with the left to the right shunt through the ductus: report of the one case. *Intern. J. Cardiol.*, 199; 49: 209-212.

[2] Kirklin J.W., Barrat-Boyes B.G.: *Cardiac surgery, morphology, diagnostic criteria, natural history, techniques, results and indication.* Churchill Livingstone: New York, Edinbourgh, London, Melbourne, Tokyo; 1993.

[3] Hoffman J.I.E., Kaplan S.: The incidence of congenital heart disease. *J. Am. Coll. Cardiol.*, 2002; 39: 1890-1900.

[4] Towbin J.A., Belmont J.: Molecular determinats of left and right outflow tract obstruction. *Am. J. Med. Genet.*, 2000; 97: 297-303.

[5] Hager A., Kanz S., Kaemmerer H., Schreiber C., Hess J. Coarctation long-term assessemnt (COALA): significance of arterial hypertension in cohort of 404 patients up to 27 years after surgical repair of isolated coarctation of the aorta, even in the absence of restenosis and prosthetic material. *J. Thorac. Cardiovas Surg.*, 2007; 134: 738-745.

[6] Niwa K., Perloff J.K., Bhuta S.M., Laks H., Drinkwater D.C., Child J.S., Miner P.D. Structural abnormalities of great arteries walls in congenital heart disease: light and electronic microscopic analyses. *Circulation*, 2001; 103: 393-400.

[7] Marx GR. „Repaired" aortic coarctation in adults: not a „simple" congenital heart defect. *J. Am. Coll. Cardiol.*, 2000; 35: 1003-1006.

[8] Hager A, Kaemmerer H., Hess J. Comparison of helical CT scanning and MRI in the follow-up of adults with coarctation of the aorta. *Chest,* 2005; 127: 2296.

[9] Connolly H.M., Huston J 3rd, Brown R.D. Jr, Warnes C.A., Ammash N.M., Tajik A.J. Intracranial aneurysms in patients with coarctation of the aorta: a prospective magnetic resonance angiographies study of 100 patients. *Mayo. Clin. Proc,*. 2003; 78: 1491-1499.

[10] National high blood pressure education program working group on high blood pressure in children and adolescents: The fourth report on the diagnosis, evaluation and treatment of high blood pressure in children and adolescents. *Pediatrics*, 2004; 114: 555-576.

[11] Borowski A., Wieteska-Klimczak A, Dorywalski T, Wyszynska T, Januszewicz P. Twenty-four-hour ambulatory blood pressure monitoring in healthy Polish children and adolescents. *Pediat. Pol.,* 1998; 73:1247-1251.

[12] Soergel M., Kirschstein M., Busch C., Danne T., Gellermann J., Holl R., Krull F., Reichert H., Reusz G.S., Rascher W. Oscilometric twenty-four-hour ambulatory blood pressure values in healthy children and adolescents. *J. Pediatr.*, 1997; 130: 178-184.

[13] Wojcicka-Urbanska B., Werner B., Godlewski K., Tarnowska A. Coarctation of the aorta in a neonate with severe clinical course and hypertensive crisis after the balloon angioplasty of the recoarctation. *Standardy Med.*, 2006; 8 (Supl) :71-74.

[14] Johnson D., Perrault H., Vobecky S.J., Fournier A., Davignon A. Influence of the postoperative period and surgical procedure on ambulatory blood pressure-determination of hypertension load after the successful repair of aortic coarctation. *Eur. Heart J.*, 1998; 19: 638-646.

[15] De Divittis M., Pilla C., Kattenhorn M., Donald A., Zadinello M., Wallace S., Redington A., Deanfield J. Ambulatory blood pressure, left ventricular mass, and conduit artery function late after successful repair of coarctation of the aorta. *J. Am. Coll. Cardioll.*, 2003; 41: 2259-2265.

[16] Trojnarska O., Szyszka A., Ochotny R., Siwinska A., Cieslinski A. Blood pressure, left ventricular mass and function in adult patients after the successful repair of coarctation of the aorta. *Kardiol. Pol.*, 2003; 59: 312-316.

[17] O'Sullivan J.J., Derrick G., Darnell R.: Prevalence of hypertension in children after early repair of coarctation of the aorta: a cohort study using casual and 24 hour blood pressure measurement. *Heart*, 2000; 88: 163-166.

[18] Sorof J.M., Portman R.J. White coat hypertension in children with elevated casual blood pressure. *J. Pediatr.*, 2000; 137: 493-497.

[19] Sorof J.M., Poffenbarger T., Franco K., Portman R.: Evaluation of white coat hypertension in children: importance of definitions of normal ambulatory blood pressure and the severity of casual hypertension. *Am. J. Hypertens*, 2001; 14: 855-60.

[20] Florianczyk T, Werner B. Usefulness of ambulatory blood pressure monitoring in diagnosis of arterial hypertension in children and adolescents. *Kardiol. Pol.*, 2008; 66: 12-17.

[21] Toro-Salazar O.H., Steiberger J., Thomas W., Rochcini A.P. Carpenter B., Moller J.H. Long-term follow-up of patient after coarctation of the aorta repair. *Am. J. Cardiol.*, 2002; 89: 541-547.

[22] Eicken A., Pensi U., Sebening W. (2006). The fate of systemic blood pressure in patient after effectively stented coarctation. *Eur. Heart J.*, 2006; www.euroheartj.oupjournals.org.

[23] De Divittis M., Rubba P., Calabro R. Arterial hypertension and cardiovascular prognosis after successful repair of aortic coarctation: a clinical model for the study of vascular function. *Nutr. Metab. Cardiovasc. Dis.*, 2005; 15: 382-394.

[24] Bold M., Neudorf U. Arterial hypertension in children and adolescents after surgical repair of aortic coarctation defined by ambulatory blood pressure monitoring. *Blood Press Monit.* 2000; 5: 163-167.

[25] Bacha E.A., Almodovar M., Wessel D.L., Zurakowski D., Erickson L.C., Mayer Jr J.E. Surgery for coarctation of the aorta in infants weighing less than 2 kg. *Ann. Thorac. Surg.*, 2001, 71: 1260-1264.

[26] Vriend J.W.J., Mulder B.J.M. Late complications in patients after repair of aortic coarctation: implications and management. *Int. J. Cardiol.*, 2005; 101: 399-406.

[27] Jenkins N.P., Ward C. Coarctation of the aorta: natural history and outcome after surgical treatment. *Q. J. Med.*, 1999; 92: 365-371.

[28] Vogt M., Kühn A., Baumagartner D., Baumgartner C., Busch R., Kostolny M., Hess J. Impaired elastic properties of the ascending aorta in newborns before and early after successful coarctation repair. *Circulation*, 2005; 111: 3269-3273.

[29] Brili S., Tousoulis C., Antoniades C., Aggeli C., Roubelakis A., Papathanasiu S., Stefanadis C. Evidence of vascular dysfunction in young patients with successfully repaired coarcttion of aorta. *Atherosclerosis,* 2005; 182: 97-103.

[30] Sehested J., Baandrup U., Mikkelsen E. Different reactivity and structure of the prestenotic and poststenotic aorta in human coarctation: implication for baroreceptor function. *Circulation*, 1982; 65: 1060-1065.

[31] Rocchini A.P. Coarctation of the aorta. In: Izzo J.L., Black H.R. *Hypertension primer: The essentials of high blood pressure*. Baltimore: Lippincott, Williams and Wilkins; 2003; 146-147.

[32] Simsolo R., Grunfeld B., Gimenez M., Lopez M., Berri G., Becu L. Long-term systemic hypertension in children after succesfull repair of coarctation of the aorta. *Am. Heart J.*, 1988; 115: 1268-1273.

[33] Vriend J.W.J., Zwinderman A.H., de Groot E., Kastelein J.J.P., Bouma B.J., Mulder B.J.M. Predictive value of mild, residual descending aortic narrowing for blood pressure and vascular damage in patients after of aortic coarctation. *Eur. Heart. J.*, 2005; 26: 84-90.

[34] Vriend J.W.J., van Montfrans G.A., Romkes H.H., Vliegen H.W., Voen G., Tijssen J.G.P. Relation between exercise induced hypertension in adult patients after successful repair of aortic coarctation. *J. Hypertens*, 2004; 22: 501-509.

[35] Johnson D., Perrault H., Vobecky S.J., Trudeau F., Dalvin E., Fournier A. Resetting of cardiopulmonary baroreflex 10 years after surgical repair of coarctation of the aorta. *Heart*, 2001; 85: 318-325.

[36] Ou P., Bonnet D., Auriacombe L., Pedroni E., Balleux F., Sidi D. Late systemic hypertension and aortic arch geometry after successful repair of coarctation of the aorta. *Eur. Heart J.*, 2004; 25: 1583-1589.

[37] Mullen M.J., Kharbanda R.K., Cross J., Donald A.E., Taylor M., Vallance P. Heterogeneousnature of flow-mediated dilatation in human conduit arteries in vivo. Relevance to endothelial dysfunction in hypercholesterolemia. *Circ. Res.*, 2001; 88: 145-151.

[38] de Divitis M., Pilla C., Kattenhorn M., Zadinello M., Donald A., Leeson P. Vascular dysfunction after repair of coarctation of the aorta: impact of early surgery. *Circulation*, 2001; 104 (Suppl. 1): 165-170.

[39] Gardiner H.M., Celermajer D.S., Sorensen K.E., Georgakopoulos D., Robinson J., Thomas O. Arterial reactivity is significantly impaired in normotensive young adults after successful repair of aortic coarctation in childhood. *Circulation*, 89: 1745-1750.

[40] Taddei S., Salvetti A. Endothelial dysfunction in essential hypertension: clinical implications. *J. Hypertens*, 2002; 20: 1671-1674.

[41] Ghiadoni L., Huang Y., Magagna A., Buralli S., Taddei S., Salvetti A. Effect of acute blood pressure reduction on endothelial function in the brachial artery of patients with essential hypertension. *J. Hypertens*, 2001; 19: 547-551.

[42] Liao D., Arnett D.K., Tyroler H.A., Ryley W.A., Charnbless L.E., Szklo M. Arterial stiffness and the development of hypertension . The ARIC Study. *Hypertension*, 1999; 34: 201-206.

In: Hypertension, Heredity and Stroke
Editor: Cristina Moratinos and Bruno Cardenas
ISBN 978-1-60741-496-4

Chapter 11

Problems of Methodology and Interpretation of Ambulatory Blood Pressure Monitoring in Children

Tomasz Florianczyk and Bozena Werner
Department of Pediatric Cardiology and General Pediatrics.
The Medical University of Warsaw

Abstract

Ambulatory blood pressure monitoring (ABPM) is a noninvasive method of blood pressure assessment commonly found as a useful tool in diagnosis of arterial hypertension in adults, teenagers and children.

For the last 11 years we have collected about 2000 ABPM recordings performed in children and adolescents. Although we have found ABPM as a very valuable method, we need to point out some important drawbacks such as: lack of standardization of recording protocol and specification of commonly acceptable normal ranges and rules of interpretation.

We perform ABPM recordings in children older than six years of age. In our opinion in these patients measurements are well tolerated, moreover the number of artifacts is small enough to qualify majority of the recordings for further analysis. Our own protocol of ABPM includes repetition of measurements every 30 minutes in daytime and 60 minutes in nighttime in the youngest patients (6 and 7 years old) and adequately every 15 and 30 minutes in older children. We believe that values of mean systolic and mean diastolic blood pressure calculated for all of 24 hours period are crucial parameters to confirm or exclude the suspicion of arterial hypertension. Nevertheless there are still some doubts how to interpret blood pressure load and nocturnal deep. We diagnose the arterial hypertension in all of those patients whose blood pressure load exceeds 25%. Children with nocturnal fall lower than 10% are qualified as a non-dippers for further observation. In contrast to a standard blood pressure measurement there are still no commonly used normal ranges. This makes a main limitation of ABPM.

Thus we postulate to prepare commonly acceptable rules of protocol standardization as well as an interpretation of recordings with a special attention to blood pressure load.

The tables of ABPM normal ranges for various ethnic groups and countries should be worked out.

Introduction

Ambulatory blood pressure monitoring (ABPM) is a commonly used tool for diagnosis and evaluation of hypertension management both in adults as well as in adolescents and children.

Compared to the standard measurement of blood pressure using mercury manometer, ABPM has a higher repeatability of the results, offering measurements during usual daily activity and sleep time as well as better predicting long-term hypertensive target-organ damage [1,2].

Our 11-year experience with ABPM in children and adolescents, totaling of 1967 examinations, allows us pointing out necessity for standardization of the methodology in order to remove currently present limitations that reduce its diagnostic value. Those include the following: lack of uniform indications to ABPM in pediatric population, ambiguity of the interpretation criteria of various parameters, and lack of standardization of technical conditions of the measurement. It is particularly important facing increasing incidence of arterial hypertension in children and adolescents [3].

Discusion

Authors of the Fourth Report on the Diagnosis, Evaluation and Treatment of High Blood Pressure in Children and Adolescents [4] highlighted the importance of ABPM in diagnosis and treatment of hypertensive disease in the pediatric population. However, the report did not define still unambiguous indications to perform ABPM, presenting only the method as a helpful tool in the evaluation of suspected white-coat hypertension, hypertensive organ injury, hypotensive drug resistance, episodic hypertension, chronic renal diseases, and diabetes.

Suspicion of white coat hypertension is one of the most important indications for ambulatory blood pressure monitoring in children and adolescents. According to other authors, the white-coat hypertension occurs in 22-88% of patients [5-7]. The analysis of our 212 ABPM records, performed form 2005 to 2007 in children suspected of hypertension, the white-coat hypertension was confirmed in 32.6% of patients [8]. Due to high risk of white-coat hypertension in children and adolescents we perform ABPM in each patient considered to be hypertensive according to the standard measurement prior to confirmation of final diagnosis and qualification for further examinations and therapy. ABPM in our division of pediatric cardiology is also routinely performed every six months in patients after surgical repair of coarctation of the aorta, patients on antihypertensives as well as in patients with prehypertension found in the standard blood pressure measurement. The determination of unequivocal indications to ambulatory blood pressure monitoring in children and adolescents seems essential in view of constantly growing population of children at risk of hypertension and resultant increased diagnostic costs; moreover, some patients poorly tolerate the examinations which is associated with limitation of daily activity and stressful situations related to carrying the device.

Ambulatory blood pressure monitoring allows evaluating a wide spread of variables describing twenty-four hour blood pressure pattern. The standard ABPM report includes mean systolic and diastolic blood pressure during the 24 hours, daytime and night-time. Some monitors also enable assessment of nocturnal blood pressure dip and systolic and diastolic blood pressure loads. No clear list of parameters that should be analyzed in children and adolescents has been established so far; furthermore it has not been determined which variables should be used as hypertension positive and negative diagnostic criteria. Most of the investigators prevent from unequivocally defining the diagnostic criteria of hypertension based on ABPM, finding increase of mean 24-hour systolic and/or diastolic blood pressure abnormal [9]. In our center arterial hypertension is diagnosed based on the ABPM if mean 24-hour systolic and/or diastolic blood pressure exceeds height- and sex-matched 95th percentile value.

An importance of blood pressure load for diagnosis of hypertension based on the ABPM was specifically risen by number of reports [9,10]. Those authors suggested that high blood pressure load allows confirming hypertension even with normal mean 24-hour systolic and diastolic blood pressures. The blood pressure load cut-off value for diagnosis of hypertension using the ABPM has not yet been defined and ranges in various reports from 20% to 50% [5,11-17]. The analysis of our own results showed that hypertension is diagnosed in each patient with systolic and/or diastolic blood pressure load at least 25% regardless of the mean 24-hour systolic and diastolic blood pressure. Patients normotensive in the ABPM with blood pressure load within 15-25% are treated as prehypertensives and non-pharmacological hypotensive methods are recommended with blood pressure measurements every 3 months.

Nocturnal blood pressure dip reflecting a difference between blood pressure during the sleep and awakeness periods is a parameter which – according to many investigators – may evidence the risk of hypertensive target-organ damage. However, it has not been established if an overnight blood pressure dip or its total lack is a consequence or cause of such complications We, similarly to other authors, define the time frame dipping using actual patient's bedtime based on patient-recorded diary of activity [3,18]. In number of studies evaluating blood pressure by means of ABPM in healthy children an overnight blood pressure dip ranged from 8% to 13% [19-21]. Unequivocal determination of normal value of an overnight blood pressure dip is difficult due to problems in the evaluation of hypertensive target-organ injuries. In our center an overnight blood pressure dip above 10% is found normal. Consequently, children with decreased blood pressure dip are considered to be prehypertensives.

A lack of homogenous reference ranges developed on large study groups is one of the most considerable limitations of ABPM use in children and adolescents. The available literature mostly references the normal ABPM values developed Soergel et al. [22] in the multicentre study involving 1141 healthy children. In our studies the reference ranges provided by Borowski et al. [23] for the Polish pediatric population were applied. These authors suggest that higher systolic and diastolic blood pressure observed in children and adolescents in our country as compared to the ones proposed by Soergel et al. may result from higher salt consumption in Poland. Considering geographic and racial differences observed in arterial blood pressure from the standard sphygmomanometer measurements, it seems expedient to develop national or ethnic tables of normal blood pressure for the ABPM in children and adolescents with respect to age, sex and height of the patients.

The principles and technical conditions of 24-hour ambulatory blood pressure monitoring in children and adolescents have not been worked out and standardized so far. It applies to age of patients qualified for the examinations, types of devices, artifact rejection criteria and frequency of daytime and overnight measurements.

In an everyday practice, oscillometric monitors, microphone recorders based on Korotkov sounds detection and devices combining the both former methods are used. Our experience includes using of both types of devices. The devices using Korotkov method are slightly more accurate but producing also higher percentage of erroneous readings which result from cuff displacement and loss of acoustic signal. Artifacts count for oscillometric devices is low, averaging to 7.8% in our material, which induced us to use those devices only. It should be noted that most of the ABPM reference values in children was developed using the oscillometric devices.

The criteria of erroneous measurements rejection from the global recording remain equivocal. In our center the measurement is classified as an artifact if systolic blood pressure is above 220 mm Hg or below 70 mm Hg, diastolic blood pressure is above 140 mm Hg or below 40 mm Hg or pulse pressure exceeds 120 mm Hg or is below 20 mm Hg. Similar standpoint was presented by Lurbe et al. [19]. The ABPM reports presented in the literature excluded form the analysis records if artifacts number was above 25-30% [19,24]. Another rejection criterion we use is a total lack of readings for over at least 120 minutes of the analysis. The number of erroneous readings during ABPM predominantly depends on patient's age and weight, type of device and site experience. Earlier (from 2000 to 2001), we rejected about 22% of examinations, while currently this number is not exceeding 4.5%. In our center ABPM is carried out in children above 6 years old; as a rule, patients at that age tolerate the examination very well. We believe the probability of obtaining a useless recording in younger children is too high to justify exposing a child to discomforts of a long-lasting examination. Exceptionally, the recordings are performed in bigger and more clam children below 6 years old. The youngest patient's age in whom a reliable recording was obtained in our clinic was 4 years. In addition, a high percentage of invalid readings is obtained in the obese children. In our opinion, it is associated with cuff displacement due to taper-shaped arm.

Programming of ABPM recorder allows setting up individual measurement frequency. The measurement protocols available from the literature presumed readings every 15-30 minutes during the day and every 20-60 minutes overnight [19,24,25]. In the most reports sleep period was defined as a time between 22:00 and 06:00 or 24:00 and 06:00, whereas awaking period – as a time from 08:00 to 20:00 [19, 24]. In our center, the number of measurements as well as sleep and awakeness periods differ with respect to patient's age. In children below 7 years old, daytime readings (08:00-20:00) are repeated every 30 minutes while the overnight ones (22:00-06:00) – every 60 minutes. In older patients the frequency of measurements is every 15 minutes during the day (08:00-20:00) and every 30 minutes overnight (00:00-06:00).

Conclusion

In conclusion it should be noted that ambulatory blood pressure monitoring is a useful diagnostic tool in hypertensive children and adolescents. However, additional investigations are required aiming in development of standards and principles of ABPM interpretation as well as in working out ethnical and national reference ranges for ABPM which should significantly improve its diagnostic value.

References

[1] Sorof JM, Portman RJ. Ambulatory blood pressure monitoring in pediatric patients. *J. Pediatr.*, 2000; 136: 578-586.

[2] Cuspidi C, Macca G, Sampieri L, Fusi V, Severgnini B, Michev I, Salerno M, Magrini F, Zanchetti A. Target organ damage and non dipping pattern defined by two sessions of ambulatory blood pressure monitoring in recently diagnosed essential hypertensive paterns. *J. Hypertens*, 2001; 19: 1539-1545.

[3] Diaz LN, Garin EH. Comparison of ambulatory blood pressure and Task Force citeria to identify pediatric hypertension. *Pediatr. Nephrol.*, 2007; 22: 554-558.

[4] National High Blood Pressure Education Program Working Group on High Blood Pressure in Children and Adolescents. The Fourth Report on the Diagnosis, Evaluation and Treatment of High Blood Pressure in Children and Adolescents. *Pediatrics*, 2004; 114: 555-576.

[5] Sorof JM, Portman RJ. White coat hypertension in children with elevated casual blood pressure. *J. Pediatr.*, 2002; 137: 493-497.

[6] Sorof JM, Poffenbarger T, Franco K, Portman R. Evaluation of white coat hypertension in children: importance of the definition of normal ambulatory blood pressure and the severity of casual hypertension. *Am J. Hypertens*, 2001; 14: 855-860.

[7] Kavey RE, Kveselis DA, Atallah N, Smith FC. White coat hypertension in childhood: evidence for end-organ effect. *J. Pediatr.*, 2007; 150: 491-497.

[8] Florianczyk T, Werner B. Usefulness of ambulatory blood pressure monitoring in diagnosis of arterial hypertension in children and adolescents. *Kardiol. Pol.*, 2008; 66: 12-17.

[9] Kennedy SE, Mackie FE, Rosenberg AR, Craig E, Kainer G. Agreement on reporting of ambulatory blood pressure monitoring in children. *Pediatr. Nephrol.*, 2005; 20: 1766-1768.

[10] Flynn JT. Impact of ambulatory blood pressure monitoring on the management of hypertension in children. *Blood Press Monit.*, 2000; 5: 211-216.

[11] Wyszynska T. Pomiary cisnienia tetniczego i interpretacja ich wynikow. In: Wyszynska T, Litwin M. *Nadcisnienie tetnicze u dzieci i mlodziezy*. Warszawa: Wydawnictwo Lekarskie PZWL; 2002; 33-49.

[12] Khan IA, Gajaria M, Stephens D, Balfe JW. Ambulatory blood pressure monitoring in children: a large center's experience. *Pediatr. Nephrol.*, 2000; 14: 802-805.

[13] Koshy S, MacArther C, Luthra S, Gajaria M, Geary D. Ambulatory blood pressure monitoring: mean blood pressure and blood pressure load. *Pediatr. Nephrol.*, 2005; 20: 1484-1486.

[14] Sorof JM, Portman RJ. Ambulatory blood pressure measurements. *Curr. Opin. Pediatr.*, 2001; 13: 133-137.

[15] Flyn JT, Alderman MH. Characteristics of children with primary hypertension seen at referral center. *Pediatr. Nephrol.*, 2005; 20: 961-966.

[16] Sorof JM. White coat hypertension in children. *Blood Press Monit.*, 2000; 5: 197-202.

[17] Lurbe E, Sorof JM, Daniels SR. Clinical and research aspects of ambulatory blood pressure monitoring in children. *J. Pediatr.*, 2004; 144: 7-16.

[18] Dimsdale J.E., Heeren M.M. How reliable in nighttime blood pressure dipping. *Am J. Hypertens*, 1998; 11: 606-609.

[19] Lurbe E, Redon J, Liao Y, Tacon J, Cooper RS, Alvarez V. Ambulatory blood pressure monitoring in normotensive children. *J. Hypertens*, 1994; 12: 1417-1423.

[20] Lurbe E, Redon J, Kesani A, Pascual J.M., Tacons J., Alvarez V., Batlle D. Increase in nocturnal blood pressure and progression to microalbuminuria in type 1 diabetes. *N. Eng. J. Med.*, 2002; 347: 797-805.

[21] Harshfield G.A., Barbeau P., Richey P.A., Alpert B.S. Racial differences in the influence of body size on ambulatory blood pressure in youths. *Blood Press Monit*, 2000, 5: 59-63.

[22] Soergel M, Kirschstein M., Busch C, Danne T, Gellerman J, Holl R, Krull F, Reichert H, Reusz GS, Rascher W. Oscilometric twenty-four-hour ambulatory blood pressure values in healthy children and adolescents: A multicenter trial including 1141 subjects. *J. Pediatr.*, 1997; 130: 178-184.

[23] Borowski A, Wieteska-Klimczak A, Dorywalski T, Wyszyńska T, Januszewicz P. Twenty-four-hour ambulatory blood pressure monitoring in healthy Polish children and adolescents. *Pediat. Pol.*, 1998; 73:1247-1251.

[24] Yetman RJ, Portman RJ. Technical aspects of blood pressure measurement in pediatric patients. *Blood Press Monit.*, 1999; 4: 155-159.

[25] Simckes A.M., Srivastava T., Alon U.S. Ambulatory blood pressure monitoring in children and adolescents. *Clin. Pediatr.*, 2002; 41: 549-564.

In: Hypertension, Heredity and Stroke
Editor: Cristina Moratinos and Bruno Cardenas
ISBN 978-1-60741-496-4

Chapter 12

Genetic Studies in Pediatric Stroke

Natasa Marcun Varda and Alojz Gregoric*
Department of Pediatrics, University Medical Centre, Maribor, Slovenia

Abstract

Cerebrovascular diseases in children are a heterogeneous group of disorders with both genetic and environmental etiological factors. Despite extensive investigation, the etiology of pediatric stroke, a potentially devastating condition, remains unknown in a considerable number of patients. In recent years, progress in the field of molecular genetics has enabled research into genetic factors. In addition, the importance of classifying stroke subtypes in children has been ascertained.

In our opinion, besides children suffering from strokes, the children of parents with premature stroke represent an important group for research into genetic factors, since early manifestations of a severe cerebrovascular event generally indicate a strong genetic basis for the disorder. Additionally, in young patients, the role of environmental factors (e.g. diet, smoking) is relatively less important. On the other hand, because of the complex nature of the disease, environmental factors have to be studied simultaneously, possibly with some of the methods enabling detection of early and subclinical manifestations of the disease process.

Furthermore, environmental exposure (e.g. infection, hypoxemia) may play a crucial role in modifying genetic expression and hence it must be carefully defined.

In light of the above, we performed a pilot study of some genetic and environmental factors in children of patients with a documented cerebrovascular accident before the age of 45 years and looked for carotid artery intima-media thickness, which represents a marker of early vascular disease.

In the future, a larger sample of these children should be studied, with careful classification of stroke and control of environmental factors. Genetic factors related to atherosclerosis and thrombosis, as well as the interaction between these factors and the role of possible environmental modifiers, should be investigated. We plan to undertake

* Tel:+38623212110, Fax: +38623312393, E-mail: natasa.marcunvarda@amis.net

such a study in the near future. The same research principle should be used in children who have suffered a stroke.

Keywords: stroke, cerebrovascular disorders, genetics, child.

Introduction

Stroke is relatively rare in children, with an annual incidence of about 2.3 cases per 100 000 children (1.2 for ischemic stroke, 1.1 for hemorrhagic stroke) [1]. In the neonatal period it occurs in approximately 1 in 4000 births [2]. Awareness of etiologic factors is essential because recurrence is possible, with serious consequences and disabilities frequently affecting the children´s quality of life [3, 4, 5]. In addition, many of conditions causing stroke can be treated, possibly preventing another stroke [6].

The risk factors for pediatric stroke are numerous and very different from those in adults [6]. In children, there is a relatively high frequency of hemorrhagic diseases, while atherosclerotic diseases found in adults are uncommon. Birth-related events, congenital heart disease, inherited arterial diseases and disorders of hemostasis are more important than in adults [7, 8]. Nevertheless, much can be learned from adult stroke trials [9].

Until recently, there have been only a few large studies of genetic and environmental risk factors, implicated in pediatric stroke development [10, 11]. In one study, a predisposing cause was found in approximately half of the children [10]. It has been shown that multiple risk factors commonly coexist in individual children, predicting a poor outcome [12]. Raised lipoprotein (a), protein C deficiency and stroke of vascular origin were found to be risk factors for recurrent stroke [11].

Before performing pediatric stroke studies, a thorough classification of stroke subtypes must be undertaken using clinical and radiologic methodology [13]. Both genetic and environmental factors should be studied since the latter may play a crucial role in modifying genetic expression [13].

The first evidence for the genetic basis of stroke came from family and twin studies [14]. A positive family history of stroke conferred a 1.76-fold risk of stroke. Monozygotic twins had a 1.65-fold increased risk of stroke compared to dizygotic twins [14]. In recent years single gene disorders causing stroke have been extensively evaluated, and in some cases, a biochemical defect and/or, a mutated gene have been identified. On the other hand, research into susceptibility genes, which might confer a small but important risk of stroke by acting alone or in conjunction with other factors, has just begun, but is progressing rapidly.

Pediatric Stroke Phenotypes

In recent years the importance of defining stroke subtypes has been ascertained. The three main categories represent ischemic stroke, intracerebral hemorrhage and subarachnoid hemorrhage [1].

Ischemic stroke is caused by luminal narrowing or occlusion of a large or small cerebral artery. In most patients, the cause for intracerebral hemorrhage is rupture of a small intraparenchymal artery. Subarachnoid hemorrhage, which occurs rarely, is usually caused by rupture of a saccular aneurysm. The etiology of intracranial aneurysms seems to be multifactorial, with an important genetic component [15]. A number of association studies have been performed investigating genetic polymorphisms involved in their formation. Candidate genes for the research were genes coding for extracellular matrix components and extracellular matrix turnover, such as collagen or metalloproteinase 9 [16].

Cerebral venous thrombosis can also be seen in childhood, although it is a rare cause of stroke [17]. The most accepted hemostatic abnormalities associated with venous thromboembolic events are factor V Leiden and factor II G20210A mutations, as well as deficiencies in antithrombin, protein C and protein S [18]. Additional acquired risk factors are also present in a high percentage of cases, particularly during the neonatal period [17].

When studying risk factors for stroke it is important to keep these different pathologies in mind. Moreover, groups of studied patients have to be as homogeneous as possible.

Monogenic Disorders Causing Stroke and Susceptibility Genes for Stroke

Monogenic disorders causing stroke probably cause only a minority of strokes. In recent years, most major gene loci for stroke have been mapped and many of the genes have been cloned. This research is important, enabling a direct diagnosis in a particular patient and providing new insights into the molecular mechanisms underlying stroke. For example, identification of the NOTCH3 gene, implicated in ischemic stroke [19], or the CCM1 gene, implicated in hemorrhagic stroke [20], revealed the involvement of cell-signaling pathways in cerebrovascular diseases, thus providing a new area for further research. In children, there is considerable number of conditions with Mendelian inheritance that present with stroke [6], although the exact mechanisms by which these mutations become pathogenic are still incompletely understood in some cases.

On the other hand, susceptibility genes are expected to be involved in many patients with stroke. Attractive candidate genes for investigation of stroke predisposition include genes presumed to be implicated in endothelial injury, thrombosis, platelet aggregation, the inflammatory response, lipid metabolism, homocysteine metabolism, and blood pressure regulation [8].

Unfortunately, candidate gene studies have produced conflicting results and have been confounded by small patient numbers, lack of controls, and technical variability. The results have also not been consistent across populations. Therefore, replication studies in a large number of patients and various populations to confirm the results of found associations are needed. In addition, there is also a possibility that another marker in linkage disequilibrium with the candidate one is causative and responsible for the found association. It is likely that no single gene is a major contributor to stroke risk, and that the relative importance of an individual gene is small, but still important.

Sickle cell anemia is the most common cause of childhood stroke, affecting up to 30% of children with the disease. The etiology of stroke is complex and poorly understood. Growing evidence suggests that genetic factors beyond the sickle cell mutation influence the stroke risk [21]. Hoppe et al. genotyped 230 children for 104 polymorphisms and showed that several candidate genes may play a role in predisposition to specific stroke subtypes in children with this disease [22]. Most recently, they confirmed the important role of TNF (-308) G/A [23].

Some HLA alleles, especially HLA-B51 have been found to be increased in idiopathic stroke patients, which might point to a genetic predisposition [24].

Disorders of coagulation have also been investigated in children [25, 26]. Inherited and/or acquired prothrombotic disorders were detected in 17% of patients with arterial ischemic stroke and in 34% of the children with cerebral venous thrombosis, respectively [27]. In American children with stroke, 63% of children had at least one prothrombotic risk factor and 28% had at least two risk factors [28]. Factor V Leiden has been the most frequently studied coagulation abnormality, with most studies establishing the positive association with stroke [29]. The plasminogen activator inhibitor-1 has also been investigated in some studies, with conflicting results being demonstrated [28, 30].

Hyperhomocysteinemia, which may be genetically determined or occurs secondary to environmental factors, has been found to be a risk factor for childhood stroke [26, 31]. A C667-T mutation of methylentetrahydrofolate reductase, which plays a crucial role in the regulation of homocysteine levels, is associated with reduced enzyme activity and is strongly associated with ischemic stroke in some studies [29, 32].

Interleukin-6, which is associated with atherosclerotic disease and is also a key mediator in the inflammatory response to cerebral ischemia, has also been intensively investigated, but studies have yielded conflicting results [33]. Other factors involved in the inflammatory response have also been evaluated, although work on the genetic basis of these complex pathways is still at an early stage [34, 35].

Elevated levels of lipoprotein (a), a low-density lipoprotein with structural homology to plasminogen, have also been recorded in some studies of childhood stroke [29]. Recently, it has been shown that the procoagulant properties of elevated alpha2-macroglobulin independently increase the risk of stroke [36].

Promoter H_2 haplotype of the plasma glutathione peroxidase, whose deficiency increases extracellular oxidant stress, decreases bioavailable nitric oxide and promotes platelet activation, has been associated with ischemic stroke [37]. Other factors involved in the nitric oxide pathway, which is one of the most potent vasodilators and a regulator of the normal vascular tone, cell adhesion, and thrombosis, are also attractive candidate genes [38].

Adhesion of red and white cells and platelets appears to be an important mechanism of endothelial damage in sickle cell disease, and may play a role in stroke of other etiologies [39]. Potential mechanisms include adhesive ligands, molecules on the red blood cells and on endothelial cell surfaces [13, 21, 40, 41].

Recently, genes regulating thrombosis, thrombolysis, nitric oxide, cytokines, vascular tone and cell adhesion have been investigated in a small group of newborns with stroke, but no differences were found compared to a control group of children [41].

It should also be stressed that there are several intermediate phenotypes, such as hypertension or diabetes mellitus, that are often involved in the etiology of ischemic stroke in adults and have substantial genetic components themselves [42]. It is believed that intermediate risk factors may be important in childhood stroke, too. In one of the studies of childhood stroke lipid abnormalities were documented in as many as one third of tested individuals, and hypertension was also present commonly [10].

Future Directions

Starting with children classified according to stroke subtypes, a thorough identification of both genetic and environmental factors modifying genetic expression should be performed. This will require carefully designed, large, prospective studies of clearly characterized and phenotypically homogeneous patients, as well as analyses of gene-gene and gene-environment interactions, which will be a complex and arduous undertaking. This will enable examination of the interaction between multiple genes and the environment, which might explain why some, but not all, at risk patients are affected. Well-defined study designs, application of newer statistical methods and computer programs, and international collaboration, since stroke is relatively rare in children, will be very important for future studies. Early vascular pathology, such as determination of intima-media thickness or endothelial dysfunction, should be verified simultaneously [43, 44]. In some studies transcranial Doppler ultrasonography has been used for detecting children at higher risk for stroke [45].

Besides children suffering from stroke, children of parents with premature stroke, i.e., before the age of 45 years, stratified according to stroke phenotypes of their parents, represent an important group for research. In this group genetic factors seem relatively more important, but control for environmental factors is still needed. We have already performed such a pilot study, but children were not classified according to stroke subtypes and other potential risk factors found in their parents, and the sample size was quite small, which might account for the negative findings of the study [43].

In the future further work in children with single gene disorders should also be performed to examine genetic interactions and environmental influences. Furthermore, there remains the challenge to unravel the exact pathophysiology of these conditions, especially the involvement of the cell signaling pathways. It is also possible that some new, as yet unrecognized, familial stroke syndrome will be found.

Traditional cardiovascular risk factors, such as hypertension or hyperlipidemia, as well as newer, non-traditional cardiovascular risk factors, such as hyperhomocysteinemia or elevated lipoprotein (a) with their genetic component and complexity should also be further investigated. Prenatal influences in genetically predisposed individuals may also be important and should be studied in future [46].

In recent years meta-analyses have emerged in an attempt to overcome the problem of underpowered candidate genes studies [47]. Although these studies have their inherent limitations, they might also be important in the future if studies are better designed and the studied phenotypes clearly described. Most of the studies published until now have been case-control studies. Other designs, such as the nuclear family approach [48], should also be used in the future.

At present, we are preparing a larger study including children of parents with premature stroke, which will take all the discussed issues into consideration. Both selected genetic and environmental factors will be studied simultaneously. At the same time, morphological and functional changes of vessel walls will be assessed. Candidate genes will include coagulation factor genes, lipid metabolism, endothelial cell function, inflammation, cell adhesion, vascular reactivity and hypertension, platelet aggregation and homocysteine metabolism.

Conclusion

Although much of the work on etiology of stroke in children has been undertaken, we are still far from completely understanding the pathophysiological mechanisms. As in other complex diseases, research into stroke is difficult because of the multifactorial nature of the disease. Multicentric studies, with a clear study design and methodological approach, as well as a well-characterized homogenous groups of included children will be required in future studies evaluating the relative importance of genetic and other factors, and their interactions. The determination of all these factors is important for better management and treatment of stroke patients and for progress in the field of primary and secondary prevention.

References

[1] Fullerton, HJ; Wu, YW; Zhao, S; Johnston, SC. Risk of stroke in children: ethnic and gender disparities. *Neurology*, 2003 61, 189-194.

[2] Lynch, JK; Hirtz, DG; DeVeber, G; Nelson, KB. Report of the National Institute of Neurological Disorders and Stroke workshop on perinatal and childhood stroke. *Pediatrics*, 2002 109, 116-123.

[3] Ganesan, V; Prengler, M; Wade, A; Kirkham, FJ. Clinical and radiological recurrence after childhood ischemic stroke. *Circulation*, 2006 114, 2170-2177.

[4] Fullerton, HJ; Wu, YW; Sidney, S; Johnston, SC. Recurrent hemorrhagic stroke in children: a population-based cohort study. *Stroke,* 2007 38, 2658-2662.

[5] Mercuri, E; Cowan, F; Gupte, G; Manning, R; Laffan, M; Rutherford, M; Edwards, AD; Dubowitz, L; Roberts, I. Prothrombotic disorders and abnormal neurodevelopmental outcome in infants with neonatal cerebral infarction. *Pediatrics,* 2001 107, 1400-1404.

[6] Roach, ES. Etiology of stroke in children. *Semin. Pediatr. Neurol.*, 2000 7, 244-260.

[7] Pavlakis, SG; Kingsley, PB; Bialer, MG. Stroke in children: metabolic and genetic issues. *J. Child Neurol.*, 2000 15, 308-311.

[8] Kirkham, FJ; Prengler, M; Hewes, DK; Ganesan, V. Risk factors for arterial ischemic stroke in children. *J. Child Neurol.*, 2000 15, 299-307.

[9] Pavlakis, SG; Sacco, R; Levine, SR; Meschia, JF; Palesch, Y; Tilley, BC; Adams, HP Jr. Lessons from adult stroke trials. *Pediatr. Neurol.*, 2006 34, 446-449.

[10] Ganesan, V; Prengler, M; McShane, MA; Wade, AM; Kirkham, FJ. Investigation of risk factors in children with arterial ischemic stroke. *Ann. Neurol*., 2003 53, 167-173.

[11] Sträter, R; Becker, S; von Eckardstein, A; Heinecke, A; Gutsche, S; Junker, R; Kurnik, K; Schobess, S; Nowak-Göttl, U. Prospective evaluation of risk factors for recurrent stroke during childhood – results of the 5-year follow-up study. *Lancet*, 2002 360, 1540-1545.

[12] Lanthier, S; Carmant, L; David, M; Larbrisseau, A; de Veber, G. Stroke in children: the coexistence of multiple risk factors predicts poor outcome. *Neurology*, 2000 54, 371-378.

[13] Kirkham, FJ. Is there a genetic basis for pediatric stroke? *Curr. Opin. Pediatr.*, 2003 15, 547-558.

[14] Flossmann, E; Schulz, UG; Rothwell, PM. Systematic review of methods and results of studies of the genetic epidemiology of ischemic stroke. *Stroke,* 2004 35, 212-227.

[15] Schievink, WI. Genetics of intracranial aneurysms. *Neurosurgery*, 1997 40,651-662.

[16] Peters, DG; Kassam, AB; Feingold, E; Heidrich-O'Hare, E; Yonas, H; Ferrell, RE; Brufsky, A. Molecular anatomy of an intracranial aneurysm: coordinated expression of genes involved in wound healing and tissue remodeling. *Stroke*, 2001 32, 1036-1042.

[17] de Veber, G; Andrew, M; Adams, C; Bjornson, B; Booth, F; Buckley, DJ; Camfield, CS; David, M; Humphreys, P; Langevin, P; MacDonald, EA; Gillett, J; Meaney, B; Shevell, M; Sinclair, DB; Yager, J; Canadian Pediatric Ischemic Stroke Study Group. Cerebral sinovenous thrombosis in children. *N. Eng. J. Med.*, 2001 345, 417-423.

[18] Chalmers, EA. Heritable thrombophilia and childhood thrombosis. Blood Rev., 2001 15, 181-189.

[19] Peters, N; Opherk, C; Zacherle, S; Capell, A; Gempel P; Dichgans, M. CADASIL-associated Notch3 mutations have differential effects both on ligand binding and ligand-induced Notch3 receptor signaling through RBP-Jk. *Exp. Cell Res.*, 2004 299, 454-464.

[20] Zawistowski, JS; Serebriiskii, IG; Lee, MF; Golemis, EA; Marchuk, DA. KRIT1 association with the integrin-binding protein ICAP-1: a new direction in the elucidation of cerebral cavernous malformations (CCM1) pathogenesis. *Hum. Mol. Gen.*, 2002 11, 389-396.

[21] Adams, GT; Snieder, H; McKie, VC; Clair, B; Brambilla, D; Adams, RJ; Kutlar, F; Kutlar A. Genetic risk factors for cerebrovascular disease in children with sickle cell disease: design of a case-control association study and genomewide screen. *BMC Med. Genet.*, 2003 18, 4-6.

[22] Hoppe, C; Klitz, W; Cheng, S; Apple, R; Steiner, L; Robles, L; Girard, T; Vichinsky, E; Styles, L; for the CSSCD investigators. Gene interactions and stroke risks in children with sickle cell anemia. *Blood*, 2004 103, 2391-2396.

[23] Hoppe, C; Klitz, W; D'Harlingue, K; Cheng, S; Grow, M; Steiner, L; Noble, J; Adams, R; Styles, R; for the Stroke Prevention Trial in Sickle Cell Anemia (STOP) Investigators. Confirmation of an association between the TNF (-308) promoter polymorphism and stroke risk in children with sickle cell anemia. *Stroke,* 2007 38, 2241-2246.

[24] Zou, LP; Guo, YH; Fang, F; Jin, H; Wu, HS; Mix, E. Evidence for human leucocyte antigen-related susceptibility in idiopathic childhood ischemic stroke. *Eur. Neurol.*, 2002 48, 153-157.

[25] Haywood, S; Liesner, R, Pindora, S; Ganesan, V. Thrombophilia and first arterial ischaemic stroke: a systematic review. *Arch. Dis. Child*, 2005 90, 402-405.

[26] Komitopoulou, A; Platokouki, H; Kapsimali, Z; Pergantou, H; Adamtziki, E; Aronis, S. Mutations and polymorphisms in genes affecting hemostasis proteins and homocysteine metabolism in children with arterial ischaemic stroke. *Cerebrovasc. Dis.,* 2006 22, 13-20.

[27] Bonduel, M; Sciuccati, G; Hepner, M; Pieroni, G; Torres, AF; Frontroth, JP; Tenembaum, S. Arterial ischaemic stroke and cerebral venous thrombosis in children: a 12-year Argentinean registry. *Acta Haematol.*, 2006 115, 180-185.

[28] Lynch, JK; Han, CJ; Nee, LE; Nelson, KB. Prothrombotic factors in children with stroke or porencephaly. *Pediatrics*, 2005 116, 447-453.

[29] Nowak-Göttl, U; Sträter, R; Heinecke, A; Junker, R; Koch, HG; Schuierer, G; von Eckardstein, A; for the Childhood Stroke Study Group. Lipoprotein (a) and genetic polymorphisms of clotting factor V, prothrombin and methylenetetrahydrofolate reductase are risk factors of spontaneous ischemic stroke in childhood. *Blood,* 1999 94, 3678-3682.

[30] Nowak-Göttl, U; Sträter, R; Kosch, A; von Eckardstein, A; Schobess, R; Luigs, P; Nabel, P; Vielhaber, H; Kurnik, K; Junker, R. The plasminogen activator inhibitor (PAI-1) promoter 4G/4G genotype is not associated with ischaemic stroke in population of German children. Childhood Stroke Study Group. *Eur. J. Haematol.*, 2001 66, 57-62.

[31] Van Beynum, IM; Smeitink, JA; den Heljer, M; te Poele Pothoff, MT; Blom, HJ. Hyperhomocysteinemia: a risk for ischemic stroke in children. *Circulation,* 1999 99, 2070-2072.

[32] Alluri, RV; Mohan, V; Komandur, S; Chawda, K; Chaudhuri, JR; Hasan, O. MTHFR C677T gene mutation as a risk factor for arterial stroke: a hospital based study. *Eur. J. Neurol.*, 2005 12, 40-44.

[33] Tso, AR; Merino, JG; Warach, S. Interleukin-6 174 G/C polymorphism and ischemic stroke: a systematic review. *Stroke*, 2007 38, 3070-3075.

[34] Iacoviello, L; Di Castelnuovo, A; Gattone, M; Pezzini, A; Assanelli, D; Lorenzet, R; Del Zotto, E; Colombo, M; Napoleone, E; Amore, C; D'Orazio, A; Padovani, A; de Gaetano, G; Giannuzzi, P; Donati, MB; IGIGI Investigators. Polymorphisms of the interleukin-1beta gene affect the risk of myocardial infarction and ischemic stroke at young age and the response of mononuclear cells to stimulation in vitro. *Arterioscler. Thromb. Vasc. Biol.*, 2005 25, 222-227.

[35] Pereira, TV; Rudnicki, M; Franco, RF; Pereira, AC; Krieger, JE. Effect of the G-308A polymorphism of the tumor necrosis factor α gene on the risk of ischemic heart disease and ischemic stroke. A meta-analysis. *Am. Heart J.*, 2007 153, 821-830.

[36] Beheiri, A; Langer, C; Düring, C; Krümpel, A; Thedieck, S; Nowak-Göttl, U. Role of elevated alpha 2- macroglobulin revisited: results case-control study in children with symptomatic thrombembolism. *J. Thromb. Haemost.*, 2007 5, 1179-1184.

[37] Voetsch, B; Jin, RC; Bierl, C; Benke, KS; Kenet, G; Simioni, P; Ottaviano, F; Damasceno, BP; Annichino-Bizacchi, JM; Handy, DE; Loscalzo, J. Promoter polymorphisms in the plasma glutathione peroxidase (GPx-3) gene: a novel risk factor for arterial ischemic stroke among young adults and children. *Stroke*, 2007 38, 41-49.

[38] Akar, N; Akar, E; Deda, G; Sipahi, T. No association between Glu/Asp polymorphism of NOS3 gene in ischemic stroke. *Neurology*, 2000 55, 460-461.

[39] Taylor, JG 6th; Tang, DC; Savage, SA; Leitman, SF; Heller, SI; Serjeant, GR; Rodgers, GP; Chanock, SJ. Variants in the VCAM1 gene and risk for symptomatic stroke in sickle cell disease. *Blood,* 2002 100, 4303-4309.

[40] Kalinowska, A; Losy, J. PECAM-1, a key player in neuroinflammation. *Eur. J. Neurol.,* 2006 13, 1284-1290.

[41] Miller, SP; Wu, YW; Lee, J; Lammer, EJ; Iovannisci, DM; Glidden, DV; Bonifacio, SL; Collins, A; Shaw, GM; Barkovich, AJ; Ferriero, DM. Candidate gene polymorphisms do not differ between newborns with stroke and normal controls. *Stroke*, 2006 37, 2678-2683.

[42] Flossman, G; Schulz, UG; Rothwell, PM. Potential confounding by intermediate phenotypes in studies of the genetics of ischemic stroke. *Cerebrovasc. Dis.*, 2005 19, 1-10.

[43] Varda, NM; Peterlin, B; Umek Bradac, S; Gregoric, A. Carotid intima-media thickness and angiotensin-converting enzyme polymorphism in the offspring of parents with premature stroke. *Acta Paediatr.*, 2005 94, 33-37.

[44] Aminbakhsh, A; Mancini, GB. Carotid intima-media thickness measurements: what defines an abnormality? A systematic review. *Clin. Invest. Med.*, 1999 22, 149-157.

[45] Kwiatkowski, JL; Hunter, JV; Smith-Whitley, K; Eatz, ML; Shults, J; Ohene-Frempong, K. Transcranial Doppler ultrasonography in siblings with sickle cell disease. *Br. J. Haematol.*, 2003 12, 932-937.

[46] Barker, DJ; Lackland DT. Prenatal influences on stroke mortality in England and Wales. *Stroke*, 2003 34, 1598-1602.

[47] Lohmueller, KE; Pearce, CL; Pike, M; Lander, ES; Hirschorn, JN. Meta–analysis of genetic association studies supports a contribution of common variants to susceptibility to common disease. Nat. Genet., 2003 33, 177–182.

[48] Horvath, S; Xu, X; Laird, N. The family–based association test method: strategies for studying general genotype–phenotype associations. *Eur. J. Hum. Genet.*, 2001 9, 301–306.

Index

A

abnormalities, 143, 144
ACE inhibitors, xii, 137, 143, 144
activation, 140, 141
adipocytes, 140, 141
adipose, 140, 141
adipose tissue, 140, 141
adolescent female, 144
adolescents, xii, 137, 138, 139, 140, 142, 143, 144, 145, 146
adult, 144, 145
adult population, 144
adulthood, 144
adults, 137, 143
African American, 144
African-American, 138
age, 138, 139, 142
agents, xii, 137
agonist, 141
agriculture, 138
alcohol, 139
aldosterone, 141
alpha, xii, 137, 140
alpha blocker, xii, 137
alternatives, 144
amelioration, 142
angioedema, 144
angiotensin, xii, 137, 141, 144
Angiotensin, 143
angiotensin converting enzyme, xii, 137, 144
animals, 140
apnea, 139
appetite, 141
ARBs, xii, 137, 143, 144
arterial hypertension, 139
Asian, 144

B

baroreceptor, 140
behavior, 143, 144
behavior modification, 143, 144
beta, xii, 137, 140, 144
beta blocker, xii, 137, 140, 144
biologic, 141
blood, 139, 140, 141, 142, 143, 144, 146
blood flow, 140
blood glucose, 143, 144, 146
blood pressure, 139, 140, 141, 142, 143, 144
BMI, 138, 139, 142, 143, 144, 145
body mass index, 146
body weight, 139, 143, 145
boys, 138

C

calcium, xii, 137, 143, 144
calcium channel blocker, xii, 137, 143, 144
caloric intake, 143, 144
caloric restriction, xii, 137, 143
cardiac output, 140
cardiovascular, 139, 143, 144, 145
cardiovascular disease, 139, 144, 145
Cardiovascular disease, 139
cardiovascular protection, 143
CDC, 138
central nervous system, 140
channel blocker, 144
childhood, 138, 144
children, 138, 139, 140, 142, 144, 145, 146
China, 138
chronic, 139
classes, 143

clinical, 139, 140
commerce, 138
community, 145
co-morbidities, 144
complement, 141
compliance, 144
complications, 139
computer, 138
computer use, 138
concentration, 141
control, 143, 144
coronary heart disease, 139, 145
correlation, 139
cortical, 141
cultural, 144
cytokines, 140, 141

D

delivery, 141
demographic, 142
demographic data, 142
denervation, 140
deposits, 141
dermatologic, 139
developing countries, 137
diabetes, 139, 143, 144, 146
diabetes mellitus, 139, 143, 144
diabetic, 145
diabetic patients, 145
diastolic blood pressure, 142
diet, 140, 142
diets, 139
diseases, 139, 142
diuretic, 143, 144
diuretics, xii, 137, 143
dogs, 139
drugs, 144

E

edema, 144
electrolyte, 143
endocrine, 139
endothelial, 140, 141
endothelium, 140
enzyme, 143
enzyme inhibitors, 143
epidemic, 138, 145
ethnic groups, 138, 140
ethnicity, 145
excretion, 140, 145
exercise, xii, 137, 142, 143, 144
extracellular, 140, 141

F

familial, 138
family, 142
family history, 142
fasting, 143, 144, 146
fat, 140, 141
fatty acid, 140
fatty acids, 140
FBG, 143
females, 137
fetus, 144
fibrosis, 141
filtration, xii, 137, 140, 144
focal segmental glomerulosclerosis, 139

G

gastrointestinal, 139
gender, 142
genetic, 138, 144
genetic factors, 138, 144
Germany, 138
girls, 138
glomerulopathy, 145
glucose, 144
growth, 138, 141
growth factor, 141
growth factors, 141
guidelines, 144

H

health, 137, 145
health education, 145
heart, 140, 141
Heart, 146
heart rate, 140
height, 142
hemodynamic, 140
hemodynamics, 140, 145
high blood pressure, 142, 145, 146
high fat, 139, 140

high risk, 140
Hispanics, 144
hormone, 141
hormones, 141
household, 145
household income, 145
human, 139, 145
human subjects, 145
humans, 140, 141
hyperactivity, 140
hyperinsulinemia, 140
hyperkalemia, 144
hyperlipidemia, 144
hypertension, xii, 137, 138, 139, 140, 141, 142, 143, 144, 145, 146
hypertensive, 138, 140, 141, 142, 143, 144, 146
hypertrophy, 144
hypokalemia, 143
hyponatremia, 143
hypothalamus, 141
hypoxia, 140

I

India, 138, 145
industrialized countries, 139, 142
industry, 138
inflammation, 141
inhibition, 140
inhibitors, xii, 137, 144
initiation, 142, 143, 146
insulin, xii, 137, 140
insulin resistance, xii, 137, 140
Interaction, 146
intervention, 138, 142
intravascular, 145
intrinsic, 141
Italy, 138

K

Kentucky, 138
kidney, 139, 140, 141, 145
kidneys, 140

L

laboratory studies, 142
lead, 140
learning, 141
leptin, xii, 137, 140, 146
lifestyle, 138, 142, 143
linear, 139
lipid, 144
liver, 139

M

males, 137
management, xii, 137, 141, 142, 143, 145
measures, 140
medication, 143, 146
medications, 144, 145
medicine, 138, 145
men, 139, 141
meta-analysis, 139, 141, 145
metabolic, 140, 143, 144
metabolic rate, 140
metabolism, 143
Mexican, 138, 145
midbrain, 141
mineralocorticoid, 141
muscle, 140
myocardial infarction, 144

N

Native American, 144
nerve, 140, 141, 146
nerves, 141
nervous system, 140
neurons, 141
nitrogen, 143
nitrous oxide, 140
norepinephrine, 140
normal, 138, 140, 141, 146
North Carolina, 138
nucleus, 141
nutrition, 138

O

obese, xii, 137, 138, 139, 140, 141, 142, 143, 144, 145, 146
obese patients, 143
obesity, xii, 137, 138, 139, 140, 141, 142, 143, 144, 145, 146
observations, 138, 139, 140

obsolete, 141
obstructive sleep apnea, 140
organ, 139, 140, 141, 146
organization, 137
overweight, 137, 138, 139, 141, 144, 145
oxygen, 145
oxygen consumption, 145

P

Pacific, 144
Pacific Islander, 144
Pacific Islanders, 144
pain, 139
pandemic, 146
parasympathetic, 140
paraventricular, 141
paraventricular nucleus, 141
pathways, 141
patients, 139, 140, 141, 143, 144, 145, 146
percentile, 138, 142
Peripheral, 141
pharmacologic agents, 143
Philadelphia, 145, 146
physical activity, 144
plasma, 141, 145
Poland, 138
population, 145
predictors, 145
pregnant, 144
pressure, 139, 140, 141, 142, 143
prevention, 145
production, 140
promote, 141
protein, 140
proximal, 141
psychosocial, 139

R

range, 139
receptor agonist, 141
receptors, 141
recreational, 138
reduction, 139, 143
reflexes, 140
regional, 138, 140, 145
regular, 143
relationship, 139, 140
renal, xii, 137, 139, 140, 141, 144, 145
renal disease, 139
renal failure, 145
renal function, 144
renin, 141
restoration, 140
retention, 140, 141
risk, 138, 139, 141, 144
risks, 141, 146
rural, 138
rural areas, 138

S

school, 145, 146
secretion, 141
sedentary, 138
sequelae, 146
series, 143
severity, 142
side effects, 143, 145
skeletal muscle, 140
sleep, 140
sleep apnea, 140
SNS, 140
social, 138
social capital, 138
socioeconomic, 144
sodium, xii, 137, 140, 141, 145
standard deviation, 138
stiffness, 141
surgery, 146
Switzerland, 138
sympathetic, xii, 137, 140, 141, 145, 146
systems, 139, 141

T

tachycardia, 144
television, 138
television viewing, 138
Tennessee, 138
teratogenic, 144
Texas, 138, 145
therapy, 142, 143, 145, 146
thiazide, 143, 144, 146
thiazide diuretics, 144
time, 139, 140, 142
transport, 138

triggers, 140
tubular, xii, 137, 140
type 2 diabetes, 144
type 2 diabetes mellitus, 144

U

United States, 137, 138, 139, 142, 143, 144, 145
urban, 138, 145
urban centers, 138
uric acid, 143
Utah, 138

V

values, 145
vascular, 140, 141
vascular disease, 140
vascular wall, 141
vasculature, 140
vasoconstriction, 140, 141
vasodilation, 140
Virginia, 138

W

weight control, xii, 137
weight gain, 138
weight loss, 142, 146
weight reduction, 143, 144
WG, 146
WHO, 137
women, 138, 139, 141